# SpringerBriefs in Well-Being and Quality of Life Research

SpringerBriefs in Well-Being and Quality-of-Life Research are concise summaries of cutting-edge research and practical applications across the field of well-being and quality of life research. These compact refereed monographs are under the editorial supervision of an international Advisory Board*. Volumes are 50 to 125 pages (approximately 20,000–70,000 words), with a clear focus. The series covers a range of content from professional to academic such as: snapshots of hot and/or emerging topics, in-depth case studies, and timely reports of state-of-the art analytical techniques. The scope of the series spans the entire field of Well-Being Research and Quality-of-Life Studies, with a view to significantly advance research. The character of the series is international and interdisciplinary and will include research areas such as: health, cross-cultural studies, gender, children, education, work and organizational issues, relationships, job satisfaction, religion, spirituality, ageing from the perspectives of sociology, psychology, philosophy, public health and economics in relation to Well-being and Quality-of-Life research. Volumes in the series may analyze past, present and/or future trends, as well as their determinants and consequences. Both solicited and unsolicited manuscripts are considered for publication in this series. SpringerBriefs in Well-Being and Quality-of-Life Research will be of interest to a wide range of individuals with interest in quality of life studies, including sociologists, psychologists, economists, philosophers, health researchers, as well as practitioners across the social sciences. Briefs will be published as part of Springer's eBook collection, with millions of users worldwide. In addition, Briefs will be available for individual print and electronic purchase. Briefs are characterized by fast, global electronic dissemination, standard publishing contracts, easy-to-use manuscript preparation and formatting guidelines, and expedited production schedules. We aim for publication 8–12 weeks after acceptance.

More information about this series at http://www.springer.com/series/10150

Regina M. Bures · Nancy R. Gee

# Well-Being Over the Life Course

Incorporating Human–Animal Interaction

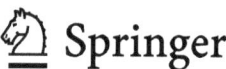

Regina M. Bures  
Eunice Kennedy Shriver  
National Institute of Child Health and  
Human Development (NICHD)  
National Institutes of Health  
Bethesda, MD, USA

Nancy R. Gee  
Center for Human-Animal Interaction  
School of Medicine  
Virginia Commonwealth University  
Richmond, VA, USA

ISSN 2211-7644  ISSN 2211-7652 (electronic)  
SpringerBriefs in Well-Being and Quality of Life Research  
ISBN 978-3-030-64084-2  ISBN 978-3-030-64085-9 (eBook)  
https://doi.org/10.1007/978-3-030-64085-9

© The Author(s), under exclusive license to Springer Nature Switzerland AG 2021

This work is subject to copyright. All rights are reserved by the Publisher, whether the whole or part of the material is concerned, specifically the rights of translation, reprinting, reuse of illustrations, recitation, broadcasting, reproduction on microfilms or in any other physical way, and transmission or information storage and retrieval, electronic adaptation, computer software, or by similar or dissimilar methodology now known or hereafter developed.

The use of general descriptive names, registered names, trademarks, service marks, etc. in this publication does not imply, even in the absence of a specific statement, that such names are exempt from the relevant protective laws and regulations and therefore free for general use.

The publisher, the authors and the editors are safe to assume that the advice and information in this book are believed to be true and accurate at the date of publication. Neither the publisher nor the authors or the editors give a warranty, expressed or implied, with respect to the material contained herein or for any errors or omissions that may have been made. The publisher remains neutral with regard to jurisdictional claims in published maps and institutional affiliations.

This Springer imprint is published by the registered company Springer Nature Switzerland AG  
The registered company address is: Gewerbestrasse 11, 6330 Cham, Switzerland

*This book is dedicated to our past, current, and future animal companions.*

# Acknowledgments

The authors would like to acknowledge the support of the public-private partnership between the Waltham Petcare Science Institute and the *Eunice Kennedy Shriver* National Institute of Child Health and Human Development. The views expressed in this book are those of the authors and do not necessarily represent those of the National Institutes of Health, *Eunice Kennedy Shriver* National Institute of Child Health and Human Development, the U.S. Department of Health and Human Services, or any component of the federal government.

# Contents

**Well-Being over the Life Course: Incorporating Human-Animal Interaction** .................................................. 1
Regina M. Bures
Human-Animal Interaction ............................................. 1
Human-Animal Interaction (HAI) and Well-Being ..................... 2
Dimensions of Well-Being over the Life Course ....................... 3
Pets as Family Members ............................................... 4
Health over the Life Course and Human-Animal Interaction ............ 4
Well-Being and Animal-Assisted Interventions ........................ 5
Conclusion ........................................................... 6
References ........................................................... 7

**Integrating Pets into the Family Life Cycle** ........................ 11
Regina M. Bures
Family Life Cycle .................................................... 11
Pets as Family Members ............................................... 13
   Young Adults and Childless Couples ............................... 14
   Families with Children ........................................... 15
   Empty Nests and Aging Families ................................... 16
Family Well-Being and Pets ........................................... 18
Conclusion ........................................................... 19
References ........................................................... 19

**Companion Animal Caregiving and Well-Being** ........................ 25
Regina M. Bures
Benefits of Companion Animals ........................................ 25
Family Caregiving and Stress ......................................... 26
Caregiver Burden ..................................................... 27
Companion Animal Illness and Loss .................................... 28
Bereavement .......................................................... 29
Continuing Bonds ..................................................... 31
Conclusion ........................................................... 32
References ........................................................... 33

ix

**Health over the Life Course and Human-Animal Interaction** ......... 39
Regina M. Bures, Layla Esposito, and James A. Griffin
Human-Animal Interaction and Health .............................. 40
Child Health and Well-Being ....................................... 40
Adult Health and Well-Being and HAI ............................... 41
Research Gaps .................................................... 42
Panel Study of Income Dynamics, Child Development Supplement
(PSID CDS) ....................................................... 43
Early Childhood Longitudinal Study—Kindergarten Cohort 2011
(ECLS-K:2011) .................................................... 44
General Social Survey (GSS) ....................................... 46
Health and Retirement Study (HRS) ................................. 46
Conclusion ....................................................... 47
References ....................................................... 48

**Human-Animal Interaction and Child Health and Development** ....... 53
Megan K. Mueller
Pets in the Developmental System .................................. 54
Social-Emotional Development ...................................... 56
Cognition ........................................................ 58
Physical Health .................................................. 59
Potential Risks and Challenges .................................... 60
Research Issues and Challenges .................................... 61
Conclusions ...................................................... 62
References ....................................................... 63

**Successful Aging and Human-Animal Interaction** .................... 69
Nancy R. Gee
Pet Ownership and Older Adults .................................... 69
  Physical Health and Exercise .................................... 70
  Mental Health ................................................... 71
  Loneliness ...................................................... 72
Interacting with Companion Animals ................................ 73
  Physical Health and Exercise .................................... 73
  Mental Health ................................................... 74
  Loneliness ...................................................... 76
Conclusion and Next Steps ......................................... 77
References ....................................................... 78

**Animal-Assisted Interactions Designed to Improve Human
Wellbeing Across the Life Course** ................................. 83
Nancy R. Gee
AAI and Preschoolers ............................................. 84
AAI and Primary School Age Children ............................... 86
  AAI and Reading/Cognition ....................................... 86
  AAI and Social Behavior Deficits ................................ 87

|  |  |
|---|---|
| AAI and Psychotherapy for Children | 88 |
| AAI and Trauma Counseling for Children | 89 |
| AAI and Young Adults | 90 |
| AAI and Special Populations of Children | 91 |
| AAI and Special Populations of Adults | 92 |
|     AAI and the US Military Personnel | 92 |
|     Equine AAI and Abused Adult Women | 93 |
| AAI and Older Adults | 93 |
| AAI in Acute Care Hospital Settings | 94 |
| Conclusion | 95 |
| References | 95 |

**Conclusion** .................................................. 99
Nancy R. Gee

| | |
|---|---|
| Social Capital | 100 |
| Cultural Considerations | 102 |
| The Needs of the Animal | 103 |
| Understanding Pet Ownership | 104 |
| Establishing the Evidence Base | 106 |
| References | 108 |

# About the Authors

**Regina M. Bures, Ph.D.** is a Senior Program Director in the Population Dynamics Branch at the *Eunice Kennedy Shriver* National Institute of Child Health and Human Development (NICHD) at the National Institutes of Health. At NICHD, Dr. Bures manages a diverse scientific portfolio in demography and population health. She has been an active contributor to the NICHD-Waltham partnership.

Dr. Bures received her Ph.D. in Sociology, with a specialization in Demography, from Brown University and completed a postdoctoral fellowship at the University of Chicago. Dr. Bures has received numerous grants and awards, including research funding from the National Science Foundation and the National Institute of Aging. Her research interests include human-animal interaction, child and family health across the life course, data science, and research methods. She currently lives outside Washington, DC, with her husband, cats, dogs, and sheep.

**Nancy R. Gee, Ph.D.** is Professor of Psychiatry, Bill Balaban Chair of Human-Animal Interaction, and Director of the Center for Human-Animal Interaction in the School of Medicine at Virginia Commonwealth University. Previously Dr. Gee served as the Human-Animal Interaction Research Manager, for the Waltham Petcare Science Institute in Leicestershire England. She has published extensively on HAI, including her most recent book; *How Animals Help Students Learn: Research and Practice for Educators and Mental-Health Professionals.*

Dr. Gee continues to pursue research in HAI across the lifespan, seeking to identify the ways in which interactions with companion animals affect human cognition, mental, and physical health. Concern for the animal's welfare and quality of life is a primary consideration for Dr. Gee, both in the Dogs on Call hospital visitation program she administers and in her various research and writing projects. Dr. Gee is a recipient of multiple grants and awards, a member of several organizational boards and journal editorial advisory boards, reviewer of HAI research grant proposals, and frequent presenter at national and international HAI conferences.

# Abbreviations

| | |
|---|---|
| AAA | Animal-Assisted Activities |
| AAI | Animal-Assisted Interactions |
| AAT | Animal-Assisted Therapy |
| ADHD | Attention Deficit Hyperactivity Disorder |
| ASD | Autism Spectrum Disorder |
| AVP | Animal Visitation Program |
| CAI | Canine Assisted Interventions |
| COSC | Combat Operational Stress Control |
| DOC | Dogs on Call |
| GSS | General Social Survey |
| HAI | Human-Animal Interaction |
| MBTR | Mission Based Trauma Recovery |
| PACK | Positive Assertive Cooperative Kids |
| PAL | Pet Assisted Living |
| READ | Reading Education Assistance Dogs |
| THR | Therapeutic Horseback Riding |
| WCC | Warrior Canine Connection |
| WHO | World Health Organization |

# Well-Being over the Life Course: Incorporating Human-Animal Interaction

Regina M. Bures

**Abstract** Human-animal interaction (HAI) is an interdisciplinary field of research that focuses on the impact of animals on human lives and the roles that they play in human lives. Drawing on the theme of well-being over the life course, we explore HAI in multiple contexts: pets as family, pet illness and aging, human health and development over the life course, and animal-assisted interventions. Conceptualizing human's interactions with companion animals in the context of the life course highlights the need for rigorous scientific methodology, improved measurement, and the application of advanced research methods to model these complex relationships.

**Keywords** Animal assisted therapy · Pet therapy · Stress reduction · Pets · Companion animals · Life course · Family life cycle · Child development · Caregiving · Stress · Aging · Health · Well-being · Bereavement · Human-animal interaction · Human-animal bond · Lifespan

> Happiness is a warm puppy.—Charles Schulz

## Human-Animal Interaction

Owning a pet is a popular choice for families. Sixty seven percent of households in the United States, about 85 million families, own a pet, according to the 2019–2020 National Pet Owners Survey (American Pet Products Association, 2019). Pet ownership has increased over time. In 1988, the first year the survey was conducted, 56% of U.S. households reported owning a pet (APPA, 2019; Insurance Information Institute, 2019). The terms pet and companion animal are often used interchangeably. Merriam-Webster (2020) defines a pet as "a domesticated animal kept for pleasure rather than utility." Companion animal, a term first used in 1897, is defined as "a domesticated animal: a pet."

---

R. M. Bures (✉)
Eunice Kennedy Shriver National Institute of Child Health and Human Development (NICHD), National Institutes of Health, Bethesda, MD, USA

© The Author(s), under exclusive license to Springer Nature Switzerland AG 2021
R. Bures et al., *Well-Being Over the Life Course*,
SpringerBriefs in Well-Being and Quality of Life Research,
https://doi.org/10.1007/978-3-030-64085-9_1

Since the late nineteenth century, the social position of pets has evolved from domesticated animals to companion animals to beloved family members or kin. This cultural shift in owner's perceptions of pets was documented in a study of pet gravestone inscriptions in the first pet cemetery in the United States, established in 1896 in Hartsdale, a village north of New York City (Brandes, 2010). Analysis of monument inscriptions in the Hartsdale Pet Cemetery demonstrated the increasing use of human names and surnames for pets, the inclusion of kinship and family terms, and, most recently, the inclusion of religious sentiments, suggesting the possibility of an afterlife for the pet.

The field of human-animal interaction, also known as anthrozoology, is a growing interdisciplinary field (Griffin, McCune, Maholmes, & Hurley, 2011). Some major topics in human-animal interaction research include the roles that companion animals play in human lives, the impact of human-animal interaction on human health and well-being, and animal-assisted interaction. Ongoing efforts to develop this interdisciplinary field have included calls for consistency of terminology and the use of more rigorous research methodologies (Vitztum, 2013). One step in this direction has been increased integration across disciplines to develop and validate measures of human-animal interaction that can be used across this interdisciplinary field.

Implicit in much of the research on human-animal interaction is the premise that relationships and interactions with companion animals have positive effects on human health and well-being. This unidirectional focus oversimplifies the complex nature of human-animal relationships and overlooks certain types of human-animal interactions. Expanding our understanding of the effects of human-animal interaction across the life course presents opportunities for researchers to develop and adapt existing theoretical frameworks to include interactions with animals and their effects on human lives.

## Human-Animal Interaction (HAI) and Well-Being

Pets can be a 'healthy pleasure' (Allen, 2003), but the research findings are mixed (Barker & Wolen, 2008; Herzog, 2011). Companion-animal owners whose pets fulfill social needs report better well-being, including greater happiness, regardless of their level of human social needs fulfillment (McConnell, Brown, Shoda, Stayton, & Martin, 2011). Companion animals can enhance psychological well-being and physical health (Hodgson et al., 2015; Wells, 2009). Animals can be protective, motivate healthy behavior change, and serve as potential participants in treatment plans. Pets may buffer the impact of stress (Beetz, 2017) or be associated with increased physical activity (Barker & Wolen, 2008). Indeed, research has shown that caring for a companion animal, such as a dog, is associated with improved well-being (Kanat-Maymon, Wolfson, Cohen, & Roth, 2020). For example, dog ownership confers health benefits, provides social support, and may increase physical activity such as walking (Cutt, Giles-Corti, Knuiman, & Burke, 2007).

To understand the effects of companion animals on well-being, research needs to focus on comparisons with non-owners, not merely between pet owners. Bao and Schreer (2016) found that pet owners were not happier than non-owners, despite having higher life satisfaction. Preliminary findings from the 2018 General Social Survey (GSS) suggest that pets owners in the U.S. may be both happier (84% versus 80%) and more satisfied with life (89% versus 85%) than non-pet owners (author's calculations, Smith, Davern, Freese, & Morgan, 2018). While Deiner and Suh (1997) define happiness, or subjective well-being, as consisting of three interrelated components (high overall life satisfaction, many positive emotions, and few negative emotions), it can be challenging to include measures of all 3 components in a broader study. Research on human-animal interaction needs to utilize common measures of subjective well-being across studies to increase the comparability of findings.

## Dimensions of Well-Being over the Life Course

Interaction between humans and nonhuman animals begins in childhood and continues throughout the life course. The life course is an individual-level construct that is linked with social processes in the family and socioeconomic environment (O'Rand & Krecker, 1990). The life course concept comprises elements including the individual life course, developmental trajectories and transitions, and established pathways (Elder & Shanahan, 2007). An individual's life course and development are shaped through patterns of growth and adaptation from birth to death. Acquiring a companion animal represents the individual's transition to pet owner and the establishment of linked lives: person and animal.

While happiness over the life course has been described as U-shaped (higher in young adulthood and old age and lower in midlife) it is unlikely that the development of well-being across the life course can be described using a single trajectory (Galambos, Krahn, Johnson, & Lachman, 2020). For example, Arnett (2018) found that midlife was stressful but, overall, it was characterized by positive well-being and many people reported enjoying their relationships with family members and pets. Evidence supports the benefits of companion animals, particularly for children and the aging population (Beck & Meyers, 1996). A review of 69 studies of human-animal interaction found significant effects across the life course on a broad range of outcomes, including improved social interaction and mood, reduced stress and anxiety, and improved mental and physical health (Beetz, Uvnäs-Moberg, Julius, & Kotrschal, 2012).

There are multiple potential explanations for the presence of conflicting results on the benefits of companion animals. The quality of the relationship with the animal may be impacted by behavioral or health issues. There may also be analytic challenges that need to be accounted for statistically: the predictors of pet ownership may also predict health status (Miles, Parast, Babey, Griffin, & Saunders, 2017). Healthier individuals may select into companion animal ownership. Health differences between pet owners and nonowners may not be solely attributable to differences in pet ownership, but to differences in socioeconomic characteristics including age, gender, race, income, and home ownership (Saunders, Parast, Babey, & Miles, 2017).

## Pets as Family Members

Companion animal researchers generally focus on the benefits of pet ownership and interactions with pets (Hosey & Melfi, 2014). The relationship between an individual and their pet is somewhat ambiguously conceptualized as the human-animal bond. While the human-animal bond may not be a substitute for human-human relationships, pets may provide other forms of social support (Hill, Winefield, & Bennett, 2020) and ease loneliness (Wissing et al., 2019). Adapting human relationship theories can contribute to a better understanding of the human-animal bond. For example, the connection between a person and their companion animal can be conceptualized as an attachment relationship, providing an emotional connection and additional support (Meehan, Massavelli, & Pachana, 2017).

Perhaps as a reflection of the complexity of individual's relationships with companion animals, a substantial majority of pet owners consider their pets to be family. In 2018, 78% of pet owners in the United States reported that they "almost always" considered their pet to be a member of their family; 90% reported "often" or "almost always" considering their pets to be members of their families (author's calculations, Smith et al., 2018). Chapter "Integrating Pets into the Family Life Cycle" (Bures, 2021) of this book focuses on the conceptualization of pets as family members and provides an overview of the roles of companion animals over the family life cycle.

Despite the overwhelming proportion of pet owners that consider their pets to be family members, the importance of the relationship between an individual and their companion animal may not be validated by social norms. The loss of a companion animal may trigger intense feelings of grief. When the norms or 'grieving rules' of a society do not recognize loss of a companion animal as a legitimate source of grief, the result is disenfranchised grief (Doka, 1999). Chapter "Companion Animal Caregiving and Well-Being " (Bures, 2021) extends the concept of pets as family to examine the impact of caregiving for sick and aging companion animals, as well as the processes of grief and bereavement associated with losing a pet.

## Health over the Life Course and Human-Animal Interaction

Over the past 10 years, progress has been made in the inclusion of pet-related measures in ongoing studies, particularly in the United States (McCune et al., 2020). Chapter "Health over the Life Course and Human-Animal Interaction" (Bures, Esposito, & Griffin, 2021) provides a broad overview of the literature on companion animals and health. It describes four contemporary population-representative studies in the United States that have included measures of pet ownership and attachment: the Panel Study of Income Dynamics Child Development Supplement (PSID CDS), the Early Childhood Longitudinal Study—Kindergarten Cohort (ECLS-K), the General Social Survey (GSS), and the Health and Retirement Study (HRS). The inclusion of these measures in the PSID CDS and the ECLS-K contribute to the measurement of the impact of pets on child well-being and development in the United States through the inclusion of measures of pet ownership in large population representative studies of children.

Children assign importance to pets in the context of their well-being (Hanafin et al., 2007). Pets are associated with children's happiness through the companionship they provide (Chaplin, 2009). In chapter "Human-Animal Interaction and Child Health and Development" Mueller (2021) focuses on the impact of human-animal interaction on child health and development and the implications for future research. Understanding the nature and quality of children's relationships with their pets has implications for public health. Child-pet relationships are complex and embedded in the child's developmental system, which includes the family, community, and broader ecological systems. Mueller provides an overview of the role of pets in the developmental system; the salience of understanding the complexities of child-pet relationships; the relationship between interaction with animals and social-emotional, cognitive, and physical outcomes; and the potential risks associated with companion animals. This situates the literature on human-animal interaction in a framework of developmental science and explores the theoretical foundations of youth-animal relationships.

Later in the life course, when the benefits of a relationship with a companion animal may be needed the most, pet ownership decreases. While more than half of individuals aged 18–70 report a family pet, this proportion drops to approximately a third for individuals aged 80 and older in the U.S. (author's calculations using the GSS, Smith et al., 2018). Analyses of data from the Health and Retirement Study (HRS) found that while pet ownership declined with age, companionship was the most common reason for owning a pet, and pet owners reported strong bonds with their pets (Bibbo, Curl, & Johnson, 2019). Companion animals can play a key role in promoting healthy active aging and may decrease feelings of isolation and loneliness (Enders-Slegers & Hediger, 2019). Chapter "Successful Aging and Human-Animal Interaction" (Gee, 2021) examines human-animal interaction in the context of healthy or successful aging, going beyond pet ownership to explore the potential impact of exposure to animals through Animal Assisted Activities (AAA) and Animal Assisted Therapy (AAT).

## Well-Being and Animal-Assisted Interventions

Animal-assisted interventions are based on the premise that exposure to companion animals provides the potential for physical and psychosocial benefits to individuals (Esposito et al., 2011; Serpell et al., 2017). In the clinical setting, researchers have reported benefits that include reductions in pain, stress, and anxiety (Bert et al., 2016), suggesting that the result is an increase in subjective well-being. Subjective well-being can influence human health (Diener, Pressman, Hunter, & Delgadillo-Chase, 2017). One way to test the effects of human-animal interaction on both subjective well-being and health is through experimental interventions designed to increase long-term well-being. Researchers could then assess the effects of the intervention on physical health. For example, interventions may include animal-assisted therapy (AAT) in a treatment plan, to assess the impact of specific types of human-animal interaction on the healing process for patients with acute or chronic conditions (Griffin et al., 2011). Chapter "Animal-Assisted Interactions Designed to Improve Human Wellbeing Across the Life Course" (Gee, 2021) presents an overview of the types of animal-assisted interventions that are currently in use, emphasizing the importance of bringing people and animals together in situations that are safe and beneficial. Well planned animal-assisted interventions often appear to be a win-win: they are popular with participants and low cost and low risk for the therapist.

## Conclusion

Bringing together research from disciplines including the social and behavioral sciences, public health, human clinical science, and veterinary medicine, the field of human-animal interaction has experienced the challenges and opportunities of interdisciplinarity. The repeated calls for consistency in measurement and methodological rigor suggest ongoing maturation of the field from multidisciplinary to truly interdisciplinary.

The field of human-animal interaction presents unique interdisciplinary research opportunities. Integrating a life course perspective into studies of human-animal interaction can serve as a tool for contextualizing its complexities. For example, as children grow up, the type and age of family pet and duration of exposure to pets and other animals may shape their human-animal interactions later in the life course. A pet can serve as a source of support that helps an individual negotiate transitions over the life course, such as children leaving home and other family life cycle transitions. On the other hand, the emotional and economic costs of a sick or aging pet can have a negative impact on an individual's well-being. Both human and companion animal outcomes are influenced by exposure to social and environmental factors that may in turn influence developmental, health, and well-being outcomes.

The prevalence of companion animal ownership around the world makes it important to understand the full range of human-animal interaction experiences (McCune et al., 2014). Given the ascribed status of pets as family members, the inclusion of measures of pet ownership and attachment in ongoing longitudinal studies is increasingly important. By applying a well-being lens to the extant research on human-animal interaction we contribute to a better understanding of the impact of human-animal relationships across the life course. The development and validation of repeated and longitudinal measures and their inclusion in population representative studies can move he field forward by facilitating research on the mechanisms that explain why and under what circumstances interactions with animals promote human well-being and positive physical health outcomes.

# References

Allen, K. (2003). Are pets a healthy pleasure? The influence of pets on blood pressure. *Current Directions in Psychological Science, 12*(6), 236–239.

American Pet Products Association. (2019). *Pet Industry Market Size & Ownership Statistics.* Retrieved October 15, 2019, from https://www.americanpetproducts.org/press_industrytrends.asp.

Arnett, J. J. (2018). Happily stressed: The complexity of well-being in midlife. *Journal of Adult Development, 25*(4), 270–278.

Bao, K. J., & Schreer, G. (2016). Pets and happiness: Examining the association between pet ownership and wellbeing. *Anthrozoös, 29*(2), 283–296.

Barker, S. B., & Wolen, A. R. (2008). The benefits of human–companion animal interaction: A review. *Journal of Veterinary Medical Education, 35*(4), 487–495.

Beck, A. M., & Meyers, N. M. (1996). Health enhancement and companion animal ownership. *Annual Review of Public Health, 17,* 247–257.

Beetz, A. M. (2017). Theories and possible processes of action in animal assisted interventions. *Applied Developmental Science, 21*(2), 139–149.

Beetz, A., Uvnäs-Moberg, K., Julius, H., & Kotrschal, K. (2012). Psychosocial and psychophysiological effects of human-animal interactions: The possible role of oxytocin. *Frontiers in Psychology, 3,* 234.

Bert, F., Gualano, M. R., Camussi, E., Pieve, G., Voglino, G., & Siliquini, R. (2016). Animal assisted intervention: A systematic review of benefits and risks. *European Journal of Integrative Medicine, 8*(5), 695–706.

Bibbo, J., Curl, A. L., & Johnson, R. A. (2019). Pets in the Lives of Older Adults: A Life Course Perspective. *Anthrozoös, 32*(4), 541–554.

Brandes, S. (2010). The meaning of American pet cemetery gravestones. *Ethnology: An International Journal of Cultural and Social Anthropology, 48*(2), 99–118.

Chaplin, L. N. (2009). Please may I have a bike? Better yet, may I have a hug? An examination of children's and adolescents' happiness. *Journal of Happiness Studies, 10*(5), 541–562.

Companion animal. 2020. *In Merriam-Webster.com.* Retrieved May 8, 2020, from https://www.merriam-webster.com/dictionary/companion%20animal.

Cutt, H., Giles-Corti, B., Knuiman, M., & Burke, V. (2007). Dog ownership, health and physical activity: A critical review of the literature. *Health & Place, 13,* 261–272.

Diener, E., Pressman, S. D., Hunter, J., & Delgadillo-Chase, D. (2017). If, why, and when subjective well-being influences health, and future needed research. *Applied Psychology: Health and Well-Being, 9*(2), 133–167.

Diener, E., & Suh, E. (1997). Measuring quality of life: Economic, social, and subjective indicators. *Social Indicators Research, 40*(1–2), 189–216.

Doka, K. J. (1999). Disenfranchised grief. *Bereavement Care, 18*(3), 37–39.

Elder Jr, G. H., & Shanahan, M. J. (2007). The life course and human development. *Handbook of Child Psychology, 1.*

Enders-Slegers, M. J., & Hediger, K. (2019). Pet ownership and human–animal interaction in an aging population: Rewards and challenges. *Anthrozoös, 32*(2), 255–265.

Esposito, L., McCardle, P., Maholmes, V., McCune, S., & Griffin, J. A. (2011). Introduction. In P. McCardle, S. McCune, J. A. Griffin, L. Esposito, & L. S. Freund (Eds.), *Animals in our lives: Human-animal interaction in family, community, and therapeutic settings* (pp. 1–9). Baltimore: Paul H. Brookes Publishing Company.

Galambos, N. L., Krahn, H. J., Johnson, M. D., & Lachman, M. E. (2020). The U shape of happiness across the life course: Expanding the discussion. *Perspectives on Psychological Science,* 1745691620902428.

Griffin, J. A., McCune, S., Maholmes, V., & Hurley, K. (2011). Human-animal interaction research: An introduction to issues and topics. In *How animals affect us: Examining the influence of human–animal interaction on child development and human health,* 3–9.

Hanafin, S., Brooks, A. M., Carroll, E., Fitzgerald, E., GaBhainn, S. N., & Sixsmith, J. (2007). Achieving consensus in developing a national set of child well-being indicators. *Social Indicators Research, 80*(1), 79–104.

Herzog, H. (2011). The impact of pets on human health and psychological well-being: Fact, fiction, or hypothesis? *Current Directions in Psychological Science, 20*(4), 236–239.

Hill, L., Winefield, H., & Bennett, P. (2020). Are stronger bonds better? Examining the relationship between the human–animal bond and human social support, and its impact on resilience. *Australian Psychologist*.

Hodgson, K., Barton, L., Darling, M., Antao, V., Kim, F. A., & Monavvari, A. (2015). Pets' impact on your patients' health: leveraging benefits and mitigating risk. *The Journal of the American Board of Family Medicine, 28*(4), 526–534.

Hosey, G., & Melfi, V. (2014). Human-animal interactions, relationships and bonds: A review and analysis of the literature. *International Journal of Comparative Psychology, 27*(1), 117–142.

Insurance Information Institute. (2019). *Facts + Statistics: Pet Statistics.* Retrieved November 1, 2019, from https://www.iii.org/fact-statistic/facts-statistics-pet-statistics.

Kanat-Maymon, Y., Wolfson, S., Cohen, R., & Roth, G. (2020). The benefits of giving as well as receiving need support in human–pet relations. *Journal of Happiness Studies,* 1–17.

McConnell, A. R., Brown, C. M., Shoda, T. M., Stayton, L. E., & Martin, C. E. (2011). Friends with benefits: On the positive consequences of pet ownership. *Journal of Personality and Social Psychology, 101*(6), 1239.

McCune, S., Kruger, K. A., Griffin, J. A., Esposito, L., Freund, L. S., Hurley, K. J., & Bures, R. (2014). Evolution of research into the mutual benefits of human-animal interaction. *Animal Frontiers, 4*(3), 49–58.

McCune, S., McCardle, P., Griffin, J. A., Esposito, L., Hurley, K., Bures, R., & Kruger, K. A. (2020). Editorial: Human-Animal Interaction (HAI) Research: A Decade of Progress.

Meehan, M., Massavelli, B., & Pachana, N. (2017). Using attachment theory and social support theory to examine and measure pets as sources of social support and attachment figures. *Anthrozoös, 30*(2), 273–289.

Miles, J. N., Parast, L., Babey, S. H., Griffin, B. A., & Saunders, J. M. (2017). A propensity-score-weighted population-based study of the health benefits of dogs and cats for children. *Anthrozoös, 30*(3), 429–440.

O'Rand, A. M., & Krecker, M. L. (1990). Concepts of the life cycle: Their history, meanings, and uses in the social sciences. *Annual Review of Sociology, 16*(1), 241–262.

Pet. (2020). In *Merriam-Webster.com*. Retrieved May 8, 2020, from https://www.merriam-webster.com/dictionary/pet.

Saunders, J., Parast, L., Babey, S. H., & Miles, J. V. (2017). Exploring the differences between pet and non-pet owners: Implications for human-animal interaction research and policy. *PLoS ONE, 12*(6), e0179494.

Schulz, C. M. (2019). *Happiness is a warm puppy.* Penguin.

Serpell, J., McCune, S., Gee, N., & Griffin, J. A. (2017). Current challenges to research on animal-assisted interventions. *Applied Developmental Science, 21*(3), 223–233.

Smith, T. W., Davern, M., Freese, J., & Morgan, S. (2018). General Social Surveys, 1972–2018 [machine-readable data file], Principal Investigator, Tom W. Smith; Co-Principal Investigators, M. Davern, J. Freese, and S. Morgan; Sponsored by National Science Foundation, ed. NORC. Chicago: NORC. NORC at the University of Chicago [producer and distributor]. Data accessed from the GSS Data Explorer website at gssdataexplorer.norc.org.

Vitztum, C. (2013). Human-animal interaction: A concept analysis. *International Journal of Nursing Knowledge, 24*(1), 30–36.

Wells, D. L. (2009). The effects of animals on human health and well-being. *Journal of Social Issues, 65,* 523–543.

Wissing, M. P., Schutte, L., Liversage, C., Entwisle, B., Gericke, M., & Keyes, C. (2019). Important goals, meanings, and relationships in flourishing and languishing states: Towards patterns of well-being. *Applied Research in Quality of Life,* 1–37.

**Regina M. Bures, Ph.D.** is a Senior Program Director in the Population Dynamics Branch at the *Eunice Kennedy Shriver* National Institute of Child Health and Human Development (NICHD) at the National Institutes of Health. At NICHD, Dr. Bures manages a diverse scientific portfolio in demography and population health. She has been an active contributor to the NICHD-Waltham partnership. Dr. Bures received her Ph.D. in Sociology, with a specialization in Demography, from Brown University and completed a postdoctoral fellowship at the University of Chicago. Dr. Bures has received numerous grants and awards, including research funding from the National Science Foundation and the National Institute of Aging. Her research interests include human-animal interaction, child and family health across the life course, data science, and research methods. She currently lives outside Washington, DC, with her husband, cats, dogs, and sheep.

# Integrating Pets into the Family Life Cycle

**Regina M. Bures**

**Abstract** Many people consider their pets to be family members yet little work to date has incorporated companion animals into the family life cycle. The family life cycle refers to the stages that individuals in a family household experience over time. Stages of the family life cycle typically include leaving home, cohabitation or marriage, childrearing, the empty nest, and widowhood. As family stages and roles change, the roles of individuals and pets change as well. Couples may be brought together by pets or may get pets as they construct a family. Unmarried and older individuals may increasingly live by themselves but have a pet. While negotiating the roles of pets in families and households can be challenging, research indicates that having pets offers benefits including companionship and stress reduction. The stages of the family life cycle and the roles of pets across those stages are described in this chapter.

**Keywords** Animal assisted therapy · Pet therapy · Stress reduction · Pets · Companion animals · Life course · Family life cycle · Child development · Caregiving · Stress · Aging · Health · Well-being · Bereavement · Human-animal interaction · Human-animal bond · Lifespan

## Family Life Cycle

The concept of the family life cycle can be used to ground the study of human-animal interaction in the family context. The addition of a pet may be considered a family transition that is experienced differentially over the life course. For example, changes in family composition and housing environment may impact a family's ability to house pets. Family change, the timing of role transitions, and pets' changing roles in families can be important considerations for human-animal interaction studies over the life course.

---

R. M. Bures (✉)
Eunice Kennedy Shriver National Institute of Child Health and Human Development (NICHD), National Institutes of Health, Bethesda, MD, USA

In the U.S., changes in family patterns and increases in longevity have made it meaningful to distinguish younger adults, adults at mid-life, and the elderly. The life course dimension that clearly reflects this distinction is the presence of children, both dependent and adult, in the home. While today married couples may spend 30 or more years together after their children leave their home, 130 years ago married couples were unlikely to survive jointly to see their youngest child married (Glick, 1955, p. 9). Since the 1970s, there has been a trend toward fewer family and married-couple households. Social and family changes, including delays in age at marriage, increases in divorce, and increases in non-martial childbearing, have led to greater numbers of single person and single-mother households. More children are likely to grow up in single-parent households. More adults are living alone, particularly those aged 65 and older (Vespa, Lewis, & Kreider, 2013).

Despite these changes in composition, families continue to make up the majority of households in the United States. The family life cycle has been used as a tool to describe families developmentally (see Duvall, 1988 for an overview) as well as from a demographic perspective (Glick, 1955). Communication and interaction among family members vary across the life course and vary by the type of social bond. The family life cycle comprises four types of social bonds: the couple (or spousal dyad), the parent-child dyad, the sibling relationship, and the relationship between friends (David-Barrett et al., 2016). Rollins and Feldman (1970, p. 21) describe 8 detailed stages:

> Stage I. Beginning Families (couples married 0 to 5 yrs. without children)
>
> Stage II. Childbearing Families (oldest child, birth to 2 yrs. 11 mos.)
>
> Stage III. Families with Preschool Children (oldest child, 3 yrs. to 5 yrs. 11 mos.)
>
> Stage IV. Families with School-age Children (oldest child, 6 yrs. to 12 yrs. 11 mos.)
>
> Stage V. Families with Teenagers (oldest child, 13 yrs. to 20 yrs. 11 mos.
>
> Stage VI. Families as Launching Centers (first child gone to last child's leaving home)
>
> Stage VII. Families in the Middle Years (empty nest to retirement)
>
> Stage VIII. Aging Families (retirement to death of first spouse).

The stages of the family life cycle reflect role variation with age: Young adults are more likely to live alone or, if married, be childless or recent parents; at midlife adults have growing children; and older adults will have completed childrearing and moved into the role of grandparent. Not all families experience the detailed stages outlined by Rollins and Feldman, and later studies of the family life cycle often collapsed stages (see Duvall, 1988; Glick, 1989). In part this has occurred because relationship and marital status changes have become more complex in modern families. Cohabitation before marriage is common. Widowhood has been postponed. Together with increases in divorce and remarriage, these changes have meant that marital status transitions are less concentrated at the beginning and end of the adulthood.

Applying this conceptualization to the study of companion animals in families, pets may serve varying roles across the stages of family development. The family life cycle is a family developmental perspective, emphasizing the roles and functions of family members; the family life course focuses on individual's transitions and trajectories (see O'Rand & Krecker, 1990). The developmental perspective can also be used to link the family life cycle and life course concepts: a period of adjustment accompanies any role change, and role changes are typically associated with transitions. The terms life cycle and life course are often used interchangeably across disciplines (see Schvaneveldt, Young, Schvaneveldt, & Kivett, 2001; Turner, 2005).

Family life cycle stages correspond to stages of the individual life course: young adulthood, family formation, parent, empty nest, and elderly. In the 1990s, sociologists merged the concept of the life course with the developmental concept of the family life cycle (Bengston & Allen, 2009). Life course theory is used to understand how individual trajectories are embedded in social pathways over time (Elder, Johnson, & Crosnoe, 2003). The concept of the family life course is used to describe the connections among individuals that may be shaped by their family background (Gilligan, Karraker, & Jasper, 2018). Similar connections to those described in the family life course may also occur between individuals and companion animals.

Non-biological families are socially constructed and may include non-human members. Fictive kin, or chosen family, are individuals who are unrelated by either blood or marriage but regard one another as family (Muraco, 2006; Taylor, Chatters, Woodward, & Brown, 2013). Relationships with pets may be embedded in family relations and conceptualized in terms of kinship (Charles, 2014; Irvine & Cilia, 2017; Power, 2008). In the case of companion animals as family, the family concept is expanded to interspecies relationships (Owens & Grauerholz, 2019) or the anthropormophism of pets (Greenebaum, 2004). Studying "pet parents," Owens and Grauerholz suggest that interspecies families may function as a nontraditional pathway to parenthood.

## Pets as Family Members

Pets can be an important component of family life (Cain, 1985; Esposito, McCardle, Maholmes, McCune, & Griffin, 2010; Mueller, Fine, & O'Haire, 2019; Soares, 1985; Triebenbacher, 2006; Walsh, 2009b). In the United States, 67% of households own a pet (APPA, 2019) and pets are often considered to be family members. According to the 2018 General Social Survey (author's calculations, Smith, Davern, Freese, & Morgan, 2018), 90% of pet owners "often" or "almost always" consider their pets to be members of their families, with women (93%) reporting pets as family more often than men (85%). These results are consistent with the 2014 Panel Study of Income Dynamics (PSID) Child Development Supplement (CDS) where 85% of primary caregivers and roughly 93% of children reported "often" or "almost always" considering their pets to be members of their families (Bures, Mueller, & Gee, 2019). Chapter "Health over the Life Course and Human-Animal Interaction" (Bures, Esposito, and Griffin, 2021) describes several large population representative surveys in the United States that include human-animal interaction questions.

Relationships with pets, particularly dogs and cats, offer forms of attachment that are associated with social and emotional well-being (Sable, 1995; Wanser, Vitale, Thielke, Brubaker, & Udell, 2019). Crawford, Worsham, and Swinehart (2006) discusses the differences between traditional attachment theory, as characterized by the Strange Situation or Adult Attachment Interview (AAI), and human-companion animal attachment. While human-companion animal attachment is distinct from human attachment, the general concept of attachment is relevant: Many of the perceived benefits of human-animal interaction are associated with companion animal attachment. For example, companion animals may be associated with strong emotional bonds, compatibility, a sense of security, and benefits to physical and psychological health (Cain, 1985; Crawford et al., 2006). A body of evidence shows that animals, particularly dogs and cats, have the capacity to develop attachment to humans as well (Berns, 2013; Udell, Dorey, & Wynne, 2010; Vitale, Behnke, & Udell, 2019).

Across the life course, pets are often considered members of an individual's family or social network and provide emotional support when coping with family life cycle changes and stress. The importance of the pet as a source of affection and attachment is related to household structure and changes over the life course (Albert & Bulcroft, 1988). Strong relationships with pets can result from accepting a pet as a primary emotional support, bonding with a pet over their personality, and having experienced transitions or change together (Reisbig, Hafen, Siqueira Drake, Girard, & Breunig, 2017). Homeless persons may consider their pets as best friends and family members, providing social support and encouraging physical well-being (Irvine, 2013). Family pet attachment is associated with both family adaptability and cohesion (Cox, 1993).

The potential for attachment and the roles and benefits of companion animals vary over the family life cycle. Based on the stages outlined by Rollins and Feldman (1970), this chapter considers the role of attachment to pets for three broad states of the family life cycle: young adults and childless couples; families with children; and empty nest and aging families.

## *Young Adults and Childless Couples*

Young adults leaving the family home are establishing themselves as individuals separate from their family of origin. Young adults living alone may have a childhood pet or acquire a new pet (or pets). The relationship between an independent young adult and their companion animal may offer insights into their level of responsibility and relationships with others. Among college students, pets function as sources of social support (Meehan, Massavelli, & Pachana, 2017). Pets may also increase the quality and quantity of social interactions (Veevers, 2016), for example, by facilitating physical activity and social interaction through dog walking and other activities. At the same time, young single adults may find it challenging to manage the financial responsibilities of a pet (Hodgson & Darling, 2011).

Attachment to pets is stronger among single individuals without children (Albert & Bulcroft, 1988). For newly married couples with no children or pets, the decision to have a companion animal may serve as a prelude for children, or it may be part of cost-benefit analysis, as illustrated by the song "I bought her a dog:"

> I met a little lady that I couldn't live without
> Much to everyone's surprise I finally settled down
> Started making payments on a house

>    tucked out in the country
>    First three years flew right by
>    Everything was going fine
>    till she threw me a curve
>    late one Friday night
>    She said: I think it might be time
>    we got started on a family
>    She swore a baby was the answer
>    to make our dreams come true
>    So I bit the bullet
>    and I did what any good, loving husband would do:
>    I bought her a dog. (Rickman, 2009)

While these lyrics oversimplify the pet decision-making process, they provide an example of the type of cost-benefit calculation that may take place. As couples create a family of their own, a pet may serve as a transition to or replacement for children. The desire for children may be triggered by loneliness or an unmet need to nurture. Attachment to a pet may reduce feelings of loneliness when pet relationships serve as a surrogate for other types of relationships, including the parent-child relationship (Krause-Parello, Wesley, & Campbell, 2014).

Perceiving a pet as a surrogate child may lead to the development of an identity as a parent (Laurent-Simpson, 2017a). Laurent-Simpson (2017b) drew on interviews of childfree companion animal owners and found that the companion animal relationship may reinforce previous fertility choices such as delaying or completely opting out of childbirth. One pathway for these outcomes was that the pets often satisfied their need to nurture without having children. She describes a level of attachment between the women and their pets that often characterized the pets as surrogate children, not just family members. Using a family life course lens to understand how couples negotiate the role of pets in families can inform research on parenthood, childlessness, and the cultural reshaping of "family" to include multispecies families.

## *Families with Children*

The role of companion animals in families evolves with the addition of children to the family and as children age. Pets can complement growing families but, they also bring challenges and potential health risks such as allergies and bites (Wanser et al., 2019). With the addition of a new family member, such as the birth of a child, pets may experience jealousy or stress. In families with young children, parental attachment to pets and time spent with them may decrease (Albert & Bulcroft, 1988).

The strength of children's attachment to pets, particularly dogs, is related to family size and type (Wanser et al., 2019). Children in single-parent families tend to have stronger attachment to dogs than those in two-parent families. This relationship is strongest for children in early childhood. For older children, no significant difference between family type and attachment to dogs was found (Bodsworth & Coleman, 2001). Children often consider their pets as siblings (Power, 2008) and may be more likely to confide in a pet than in a human sibling. They also report fewer conflicts with their pets than with other siblings (Cassels, White, Gee, & Hughes, 2017).

As children transition to adolescence, caring for pets often increases. Early adolescents report gaining responsibility, friendship, and knowledge from their pet (Covert, Whiren, Keith, & Nelson, 1985). Hawkins and Williams (2017) found strong associations between pet attachment and caring behavior among 7–12 year olds. The researchers suggest that encouraging children to care for pets may contribute to positive outcomes for both the children, through better well-being, and the pets, through better care. Young adolescents in families with dogs reported more overall satisfaction and companionship with their pets than did owners of other pets (Cassels et al., 2017).

The findings on the impact of pets on adolescents and their families is mixed. This may reflect other transitions that occur during this period as well as transitions in the types of family pets. Marsa-Sambola et al. (2016) analyze a large sample of 11-to 15-year-old adolescents from England, Scotland, and Wales and describe a number of sociodemographic differences in pet ownership. Older adolescents were more likely to have dogs and less likely to have smaller pets such as reptiles, fish, amphibians, or small mammals. Family characteristics are also associated with having a pet and type of pet. In an Australian study, older adolescents (mean age 15.9) were found to have little interaction with pets, and having a pet had no significant health benefits (Mathers, Canterford, Olds, Waters, & Wake, 2010). Other research on rural adolescents suggests that companion animals may reduce adolescent loneliness and facilitate social support networks (Black, 2012).

For adolescents, pets offer a non-judgmental companion and the opportunity to share affection (Damour, 2019). Attachment to pets such as cats and dogs is associated with improved quality of life and interactions with parents and friends (Marsa-Sambola et al., 2017). More research across adolescence is needed to better understand how relationships with pets mature (Muldoon, Williams, & Currie, 2019). The impact of companion animals on child development is discussed in greater detail in chapter "Human-Animal Interaction and Child Health and Development" (Mueller, 2021).

## *Empty Nests and Aging Families*

As individuals and families age, the potential health benefits of pets, or *zooeyia* (Hodgson et al., 2015), may increase. While the empty nest is associated with generally positive effects on well-being and marital satisfaction (Davis, Kim, & Fingerman, 2016; White & Edwards, 1990), physical health may begin to decline at midlife (see Brim, Ryff, & Kessler, 2019). Broader definitions of family are associated with greater social-needs fulfillment (Buchanan & McConnell, 2017). While Buchanan and McConnell did not focus explicitly on pets as family, the idea that families can help to buffer stress is consistent with much of the literature on pets and socialization.

Companion animals meet relational needs for consistent, reliable bonds and may facilitate transitions through disruptive life changes (Walsh, 2009a). As children leave the home, pets may offer the companionship similar to that of other family members. Companionship has been identified as one benefit of owning a pet (Garrity & Stallones, 1998). Age, having no children, or living in a household of one or two people has sometimes been associated with a stronger companion animal bond (Cohen, 2002).

Pets can serve multiple roles for individuals with long term chronic conditions such as diabetes or chronic heart disease. Relationships with pets may contribute to stress reduction by reducing cardiovascular reactivity (Allen, Blascovich, & Mendes, 2002). By helping individuals manage emotions, pets can help improve disease management (Brooks et al., 2013). For chronically ill older adults, a pet can serve as an important companion and as a motivating force for getting out of the hospital, returning home, and being active. Ryan and Ziebland (2015) found that the strength of the human-animal bond was recognized by family members and care providers who, in some cases, brought the patient's pet to the hospital setting.

For caregivers, pets may provide support and stress relief but at a cost. In a study of dementia caregivers, pets provided relief from stress but posed an additional care burden. An additional stressor could be the relationship of the caregiver's spouse with the pet, which often changed as a result of disease progression (Connell, Janevic, Solway, & McLaughlin, 2007). Pets may have stronger health benefits for single individuals (Allen, 2003). For example, dogs may take on the role of a partner when it comes to emotional disclosures (Evans-Wilday, Hall, Hogue, & Mills, 2018). Elderly dog owners tend to be less socially isolated than elderly individuals without pets (Hajek & König, 2019).

For older individuals transitioning to residential care, the exclusion of companion animals makes the transition a double loss of both home and family member that can have a negative impact on their well-being (Fox & Ray, 2019). Pets provide support and companionship and should be considered as part of individual care planning (McColgan & Schofield, 2007).

Companion animals can play an important role in well-being in later life (Walsh, 2009a). For the elderly, who may face the loss of a spouse/partner or experience changes in health status and other disruptions, a pet can be an important constant that helps maintain the activities of daily life (Fox & Ray, 2019). Pets often supply comfort and reduce feelings of loneliness during adversity or stressful family transitions such as divorce or bereavement (Sable, 1995). Chapter "Successful Aging and Human-Animal Interaction" (Gee, 2021) discusses this in more detail.

## Family Well-Being and Pets

Viewing a companion animal as a family member is positively associated with better well-being (McConnell, Paige Lloyd, & Humphrey, 2019). Pets play a complementary role to humans in the family. The identification of pets as family members and the related family narratives reflect the functions of pets in a household (Tovares, 2010). For situations where human companionship is lacking, pets may help to fill this gap (Cohen, 2002).

Pets can provide emotional support during periods of stress (Melson & Fin, 2015). Pets can also serve as a protective buffer between family stress and individuals, particularly children. These are important elements of family resilience and helping families deal with stressful situations (Walsh, 2016). For example, in a sample of families with an autistic child, the benefits of pet dog ownership persisted 2–3 years later at follow-up and included reduced family difficulties and parental stress (Hall, Wright, Hames, Mills, & PAWS Team, 2016). Linder, Sacheck, Noubary, Nelson, and Freeman (2017) found greater average attachment to dogs and lower perceived social support from peers and parents among children aged 8–13 who are overweight or obese. This suggests that dogs may serve a larger role in the social support networks of overweight/obese children's than for healthy weight children.

Children's experiences with animals are an important part of the evaluation process for professionals who encounter children exposed to, or at risk for, family violence (McDonald et al., 2018). The well-being of family and pets is frequently intertwined in cases of interpersonal violence, which is often linked to animal abuse (Flynn, 2011). Flynn (2000a) noted that family scholars typically overlooked the issue of violence to animals despite the potential for negative developmental consequences: a link with interpersonal violence, the potential for animal abuse, and the abuse of animals as a marker for family violence.

While pets can serve as important sources of emotional support in abuse situations, they can also serve as scapegoats (Flynn, 2000b). Concerns for the pets' well-being may cause women to postpone seeking assistance or shelter. Women whose pets had been threatened or harmed were more likely to report that their pets had influenced their decision to leave or stay (Faver & Strand, 2003). Some victims report that pets provide their main source of support, and that they choose to stay in an abusive relationship because shelters do not allow pets (Newberry, 2017).

Children exposed to family violence are at increased risk of exposure to companion animal maltreatment. This childhood exposure may be associated with the development of childhood and adult psychopathy (McDonald et al., 2017). Overall, children exposed to domestic violence experience both risks and benefits associated with pets in the household (Collins et al., 2018; McDonald et al., 2017) and often have high levels of positive engagement with pets (McDonald et al., 2018).

High levels of positive engagement with a family pet moderate the effects of exposure to violence on negative psychological outcomes (Hawkins et al., 2019). More research is needed to understand the separate and cumulative effects of both interpersonal violence and animal maltreatment in the family setting and the implications those have for family well-being.

## Conclusion

Human beings have interacted with animals for thousands of years. The relationships between humans and companion animals may be characterized by a strong emotional attachment or a working partnership. Pets, like dogs, may serve as companions or offer security and serve as hunting partner. While many individuals consider their pets to be family members, not all families will have pets or want them. There may be differing attitudes about pets within a family. Pets may cause conflict in families or bring families closer together. As with inter-personal relationships, the role of companion animals varies over the family life cycle.

The concept of the family life cycle can be used as a tool to ground the study of human-animal interaction in the family context. The changing roles of companion animals in families can be important considerations for human-animal interaction studies over the life course. Incorporating the roles and functions of pets into the family life cycle explicitly links companion animals to family change and transitions. In this context, the addition, or loss, of a pet may be considered a family transition that is experienced differentially over the both the family life cycle and an individual's life course.

Distinguishing between the family life cycle and the family life course draws attention to the need for the inclusion of measures of companion animals and attachment in long-term longitudinal studies. Without such data, researchers cannot tell the full story of human-companion animal interaction over the family life cycle. In addition to variation over time, such studies would shed light on variation in family and companion animal ownership patterns by race, ethnicity, and culture. These factors may shape both patterns of pet ownership, such as number of or types of pets, as well as attitudes about the role of companion animals in families. Future research on families and companion animals should include diverse, longitudinal, population representative samples when possible.

## References

Albert, A., & Bulcroft, K. (1988). Pets, families, and the life course. *Journal of Marriage and the Family, 50*(2), 543–552.

Allen, K. (2003). Are pets a healthy pleasure? The influence of pets on blood pressure. *Current Directions in Psychological Science, 12*(6), 236–239.

Allen, K., Blascovich, J., & Mendes, W. B. (2002). Cardiovascular reactivity and the presence of pets, friends, and spouses: The truth about cats and dogs. *Psychosomatic Medicine, 64*(5), 727–739.

American Pet Products Association. (2019). *Pet Industry Market Size & Ownership Statistics*. Retrieved October 15, 2019, from https://www.americanpetproducts.org/press_industrytrends.asp.

Bengtson, V. L., & Allen, K. R. (2009). The life course perspective applied to families over time. In *Sourcebook of family theories and methods* (pp. 469–504). Boston, MA: Springer.

Berns, G. (2013, October 5). Dogs are people, too. *The New York Times*.

Black, K. (2012). The relationship between companion animals and loneliness among rural adolescents. *Journal of Pediatric Nursing, 27*(2), 103–112.

Bodsworth, W., & Coleman, G. J. (2001). Child-companion animal attachment bonds in single and two-parent families. *Anthrozoös, 14*(4), 216–223.

Brim, O. G., Ryff, C. D., & Kessler, R. C. (Eds.). (2019). *How healthy are we? A national study of well-being at midlife*. Chicago: University of Chicago Press.

Brooks, H. L., Rogers, A., Kapadia, D., Pilgrim, J., Reeves, D., & Vassilev, I. (2013). Creature comforts: Personal communities, pets and the work of managing a long-term condition. *Chronic Illness, 9*(2), 87–102.

Buchanan, T. M., & McConnell, A. R. (2017). Family as a source of support under stress: Benefits of greater breadth of family inclusion. *Self and Identity, 16*(1), 97–122.

Bures, R. M., Mueller, M. K., & Gee, N. R. (2019). Measuring human-animal attachment in a large US survey: Two brief measures for children and their primary caregivers. *Frontiers in Public Health, 7*, 107.

Cain, A. O. (1985). Pets as family members. *Marriage & Family Review, 8*(3–4), 5–10.

Cassels, M. T., White, N., Gee, N., & Hughes, C. (2017). One of the family? Measuring young adolescents' relationships with pets and siblings. *Journal of Applied Developmental Psychology, 49*, 12–20.

Charles, N. (2014). 'Animals just love you as you are': Experiencing kinship across the species barrier. *Sociology, 48*(4), 715–730.

Cohen, S. P. (2002). Can pets function as family members? *Western Journal of Nursing Research, 24*(6), 621–638.

Collins, E. A., Cody, A. M., McDonald, S. E., Nicotera, N., Ascione, F. R., & Williams, J. H. (2018). A template analysis of intimate partner violence survivors' experiences of animal maltreatment: Implications for safety planning and intervention. *Violence against women, 24*(4), 452–476.

Connell, C. M., Janevic, M. R., Solway, E., & McLaughlin, S. J. (2007). Are pets a source of support or added burden for married couples facing dementia? *Journal of Applied Gerontology, 26*(5), 472–485.

Covert, A. M., Whiren, A. P., Keith, J., & Nelson, C. (1985). Pets, early adolescents, and families. *Marriage & Family Review, 8*(3–4), 95–108.

Cox, R. P. (1993). The human/animal bond as a correlate of family functioning. *Clinical Nursing Research, 2*(2), 224–231.

Crawford, E. K., Worsham, N. L., & Swinehart, E. R. (2006). Benefits derived from companion animals, and the use of the term "attachment". *Anthrozoös, 19*(2), 98–112.

Damour, L. (2019, July 4). What do teenagers need? Ask the family dog. *New York Times*. Retrieved from https://www.nytimes.com/2019/07/04/well/family/teenagers-pets-dogs.html.

David-Barrett, T., Kertesz, J., Rotkirch, A., Ghosh, A., Bhattacharya, K., Monsivais, D., & Kaski, K. (2016). Communication with family and friends across the life course. *PLoS ONE, 11*(11), e0165687.

Davis, E. M., Kim, K., & Fingerman, K. L. (2016). Is an empty nest best? Coresidence with adult children and parental marital quality before and after the great recession. *The Journals of Gerontology: Series B, 73*(3), 372–381.

Duvall, E. M. (1988). Family development's first forty years. *Family Relations, 37*(1), 127–134.

Elder, G. H., Johnson, M. K., & Crosnoe, R. (2003). The emergence and development of life course theory. In *Handbook of the life course* (pp. 3–19). Boston, MA: Springer.

Esposito, L. E., McCardle, P., Maholmes, V., McCune, S., & Griffin, J. A. (2010). Introduction. In P. McCardle, M. McCune, J. A. Griffin, L., Esposito, & L. Freund (Eds.), *Animals in our lives:*

*Human-animal interaction in family, community, & therapeutic settings* (pp. 1–5). Baltimore: Brookes.

Evans-Wilday, A. S., Hall, S. S., Hogue, T. E., & Mills, D. S. (2018). Self-disclosure with dogs: Dog owners' and non-dog owners' willingness to disclose emotional topics. *Anthrozoös, 31*(3), 353–366.

Faver, C. A., & Strand, E. B. (2003). To leave or to stay? Battered women's concern for vulnerable pets. *Journal of interpersonal violence, 18*(12), 1367–1377.

Flynn, C. P. (2000a). Why family professionals can no longer ignore violence toward animals. *Family Relations, 49*(1), 87–95.

Flynn, C. P. (2000b). Woman's best friend: Pet abuse and the role of companion animals in the lives of battered women. *Violence Against Women, 6*(2), 162–177.

Flynn, C. P. (2011). Examining the links between animal abuse and human violence. *Crime, Law and Social Change, 55*(5), 453–468.

Fox, M., & Ray, M. (2019). No pets allowed? Companion animals, older people and residential care. *Medical Humanities, 45*(2), 211–222.

Garrity, T. F., & Stallones, L. (1998). Effects of pet contact on human well-being: Review of recent research. In C. C. Wilson & D. C. Turner (Eds.), *Companion animals in human health* (pp. 3–22). Thousand Oaks, CA: Sage.

Gilligan, M., Karraker, A., & Jasper, A. (2018). Linked lives and cumulative inequality: A multigenerational family life course framework. *Journal of Family Theory & Review, 10*(1), 111–125.

Glick, P. C. (1955). The life cycle of the family. *Marriage and Family Living, 17*(1), 3–9.

Glick, P. C. (1989). The family life cycle and social change. *Family Relations, 38*(2), 123–129.

Greenebaum, J. (2004). It's a dog's life: Elevating status from pet to"fur baby" at yappy hour. *Society & Animals, 12*(2), 117–135.

Hall, S. S., Wright, H. F., Hames, A., Mills, D. S., & PAWS Team. (2016). The long-term benefits of dog ownership in families with children with autism. *Journal of Veterinary Behavior, 13*, 46–54.

Hawkins, R., & Williams, J. (2017). Childhood attachment to pets: Associations between pet attachment, attitudes to animals, compassion, and humane behaviour. *International Journal of Environmental Research and Public Health, 14*(5), 490.

Hawkins, R. D., McDonald, S. E., O'Connor, K., Matijczak, A., Ascione, F. R., & Williams, J. H. (2019). Exposure to intimate partner violence and internalizing symptoms: The moderating effects of positive relationships with pets and animal cruelty exposure. *Child Abuse and Neglect, 98*, 104166.

Hajek, A., & König, H. H. (2019). How do cat owners, dog owners and individuals without pets differ in terms of psychosocial outcomes among individuals in old age without a partner? *Aging & Mental Health*, 1–7.

Hodgson, K., & Darling, M. (2011). Pets in the family: Practical approaches. *Journal of the American Animal Hospital Association, 47*(5), 299–305.

Hodgson, K., Barton, L., Darling, M., Antao, V., Kim, F. A., & Monavvari, A. (2015). Pets' impact on your patients' health: Leveraging benefits and mitigating risk. *The Journal of the American Board of Family Medicine, 28*(4), 526–534.

Irvine, L. (2013). Animals as lifechangers and lifesavers: Pets in the redemption narratives of homeless people. *Journal of Contemporary Ethnography, 42*(1), 3–30.

Irvine, L., & Cilia, L. (2017). More-than-human families: Pets, people, and practices in multispecies households. *Sociology Compass, 11*(2), e12455.

Krause-Parello, C. A., Wesley, Y., & Campbell, M. (2014). Examining pet attitude in relationship to loneliness and parenthood motivation in pet-owning adults. *Health, 6*, 598–606.

Laurent-Simpson, A. (2017a, September). Considering alternate sources of role identity: Childless parents and their animal "kids". *Sociological Forum, 32*(3), 610–634.

Laurent-Simpson, A. (2017b). "They Make Me Not Wanna Have a Child": Effects of Companion Animals on Fertility Intentions of the Childfree. *Sociological Inquiry, 87*(4), 586–607.

Linder, D. E., Sacheck, J. M., Noubary, F., Nelson, M. E., & Freeman, L. M. (2017). Dog attachment and perceived social support in overweight/obese and healthy weight children. *Preventive Medicine Reports, 6,* 352–354.

Marsa-Sambola, F., Williams, J., Muldoon, J., Lawrence, A., Connor, M., Roberts, C., … Currie, C. (2016). Sociodemographics of pet ownership among adolescents in Great Britain: Findings from the HBSC Study in England, Scotland, and Wales. *Anthrozoös, 29*(4), 559–580.

Marsa-Sambola, F., Williams, J., Muldoon, J., Lawrence, A., Connor, M., & Currie, C. (2017). Quality of life and adolescents' communication with their significant others (mother, father, and best friend): The mediating effect of attachment to pets. *Attachment & Human Development, 19*(3), 278–297.

Mathers, M., Canterford, L., Olds, T., Waters, E., & Wake, M. (2010). Pet ownership and adolescent health: Cross-sectional population study. *Journal of Paediatrics and Child Health, 46*(12), 729–735.

McColgan, G., & Schofield, I. (2007). The importance of companion animal relationships in the lives of older people. *Nursing Older People, 19*(1), 21–23.

McConnell, A. R., Paige Lloyd, E., & Humphrey, B. T. (2019). We are family: Viewing Pets as Family Members Improves Wellbeing. *Anthrozoös, 32*(4), 459–470.

McDonald, S. E., Dmitrieva, J., Shin, S., Hitti, S. A., Graham-Bermann, S. A., Ascione, F. R., & Williams, J. H. (2017). The role of callous/unemotional traits in mediating the association between animal abuse exposure and behavior problems among children exposed to intimate partner violence. *Child Abuse and Neglect, 72,* 421–432.

McDonald, S. E., Cody, A. M., Booth, L. J., Peers, J. R., Luce, C. O. C., Williams, J. H., & Ascione, F. R. (2018). Animal cruelty among children in violent households: Children's explanations of their behavior. *Journal of Family Violence, 33*(7), 469–480.

Meehan, M., Massavelli, B., & Pachana, N. (2017). Using attachment theory and social support theory to examine and measure pets as sources of social support and attachment figures. *Anthrozoös, 30*(2), 273–289.

Melson, G. F., & Fine, A. H. (2015). Animals in the lives of children. In *Handbook on animal-assisted therapy* (pp. 179–194). San Diego: Academic Press.

Mueller, M. K., Fine, A. H., & O'Haire, M. E. (2019). Understanding the role of human-animal interaction in the family context. In A. H. Fine (Ed.), *Handbook on animal-assisted therapy: Theoretical foundations and guidelines for applying animal assisted interventions* (5th ed., pp. 351–362). Amsterdam: Elsevier.

Muldoon, J. C., Williams, J. M., & Currie, C. (2019). Differences in boys' and girls' attachment to pets in early-mid adolescence. *Journal of Applied Developmental Psychology, 62,* 50–58.

Muraco, A. (2006). Intentional families: Fictive kin ties between cross-gender, different sexual orientation friends. *Journal of Marriage and Family, 68*(5), 1313–1325.

Newberry, M. (2017). Pets in danger: Exploring the link between domestic violence and animal abuse. *Aggression and Violent Behavior, 34,* 273–281.

O'Rand, A. M., & Krecker, M. L. (1990). Concepts of the life cycle: Their history, meanings, and uses in the social sciences. *Annual Review of Sociology, 16*(1), 241–262.

Owens, N., & Grauerholz, L. (2019). Interspecies Parenting: How Pet Parents Construct Their Roles. *Humanity & Society, 43*(2), 96–119.

Power, E. (2008). Furry families: Making a human–dog family through home. *Social and Cultural Geography, 9*(5), 535–555.

Reisbig, A. M., Hafen, M., Jr., Siqueira Drake, A. A., Girard, D., & Breunig, Z. B. (2017). Companion animal death: A qualitative analysis of relationship quality, loss, and coping. *OMEGA-Journal of Death and Dying, 75*(2), 124–150.

Rickman, B. (2009). I bought her a dog [Song]. On Young Man, Old Soul. Rural Rhythm.

Rollins, B. C., & Feldman, H. (1970). Marital satisfaction over the family life cycle. *Journal of Marriage and the Family, 32,* 20–28.

Ryan, S., & Ziebland, S. (2015). On interviewing people with pets: Reflections from qualitative research on people with long-term conditions. *Sociology of Health & Illness, 37*(1), 67–80.

Sable, P. (1995). Pets, attachment, and well-being across the life cycle. *Social Work, 40*(3), 334–341.

Schvaneveldt, P. L., Young, M. H., Schvaneveldt, J. D., & Kivett, V. R. (2001). Interaction of people and pets in the family setting: A life course perspective. *Journal of Teaching in Marriage & Family, 1*(2), 34–51.

Smith, T. W., Davern, M., Freese, J., & Morgan, S. (2018). *General Social Surveys, 1972–2018 [machine-readable data file]*, Principal Investigator, Tom W. Smith; Co-Principal Investigators, M. Davern, J. Freese, and S. Morgan; Sponsored by National Science Foundation, ed. NORC. Chicago: NORC. NORC at the University of Chicago [producer and distributor]. Data accessed from the GSS Data Explorer website at gssdataexplorer.norc.org.

Soares, C. J. (1985). The companion animal in the context of the family system. *Marriage & Family Review, 8*(3–4), 49–62.

Taylor, R. J., Chatters, L. M., Woodward, A. T., & Brown, E. (2013). Racial and ethnic differences in extended family, friendship, fictive kin, and congregational informal support networks. *Family Relations, 62*(4), 609–624.

Tovares, A. V. (2010). All in the family: Small stories and narrative construction of a shared family identity that includes pets. *Narrative Inquiry, 20*(1), 1–19.

Triebenbacher, S. L. (2006). The companion animal within the family system: The manner in which animals enhance life within the home. In *Handbook on animal-assisted therapy* (pp. 357–374). San Diego: Academic Press.

Turner, W. G. (2005). The role of companion animals throughout the family life cycle. *Journal of Family Social Work, 9*(4), 11–21.

Udell, M. A., Dorey, N. R., & Wynne, C. D. (2010). What did domestication do to dogs? A new account of dogs' sensitivity to human actions. *Biological Reviews, 85*(2), 327–345.

Vespa, J., Lewis, J., M., & Kreider, R., M. (2013). America's Families and Living Arrangements: 2012. In *Current Population Reports* (pp. 20–570). Washington, DC: U.S. Census Bureau.

Veevers, J. E. (2016). The social meanings of pets: Alternative roles for companion animals. In *Pets and the Family* (pp. 11–30). Routledge.

Vitale, K. R., Behnke, A. C., & Udell, M. A. (2019). Attachment bonds between domestic cats and humans. *Current Biology, 29*(18), R864–R865.

Walsh, F. (2009a). Human-animal bonds I: The relational significance of companion animals. *Family Process, 48*(4), 462–480.

Walsh, F. (2009b). Human-Animal bonds II: The role of pets in family systems and family therapy. *Family Process, 48*(4), 481–499.

Walsh, F. (2016). Family resilience: A developmental systems framework. *European Journal of Developmental Psychology, 13*(3), 313–324.

Wanser, S. H., Vitale, K. R., Thielke, L. E., Brubaker, L., & Udell, M. A. (2019). Spotlight on the psychological basis of childhood pet attachment and its implications. *Psychology Research and Behavior Management, 12,* 469. https://www.ncbi.nlm.nih.gov/pmc/articles/PMC6610550/.

White, L., & Edwards, J. N. (1990). Emptying the nest and parental well-being: An analysis of national panel data. *American Sociological Review*, 235–242.


**Regina M. Bures, Ph.D.** is a Senior Program Director in the Population Dynamics Branch at the *Eunice Kennedy Shriver* National Institute of Child Health and Human Development (NICHD) at the National Institutes of Health. At NICHD, Dr. Bures manages a diverse scientific portfolio in demography and population health. She has been an active contributor to the NICHD-Waltham partnership. Dr. Bures received her Ph.D. in Sociology, with a specialization in Demography, from Brown University and completed a postdoctoral fellowship at the University of Chicago. Dr. Bures has received numerous grants and awards, including research funding from the National Science Foundation and the National Institute of Aging. Her research interests include human-animal interaction, child and family health across the life course, data science, and research methods. She currently lives outside Washington, DC, with her husband, cats, dogs, and sheep.

# Companion Animal Caregiving and Well-Being

Regina M. Bures

**Abstract** Much of the research on human-animal interaction measures the impact of the presence of a companion animal or the interaction with a specific type of animal on human well-being. Little attention has been given to measurement of the animal's well-being and the impact of a companion animal's declining health or death on the human caregiver. Caring for a sick or aging animal can be time consuming, emotionally draining, and financially expensive. Some of the conflicting results in the human-animal interaction literature may be accounted for by such factors as the level of attachment to the animal, involvement with the animal, and in particular the age and health status of the animal. Research challenges and the need to recognize and measure the effects of companion animal caregiving are discussed, particularly in the context of chronic illness, aging, and bereavement.

**Keywords** Animal assisted therapy · Pet therapy · Stress reduction · Pets · Companion animals · Life course · Family life cycle · Child development · Caregiving · Stress · Aging · Health · Well-being · Bereavement · Human-animal interaction · Human-animal bond · Lifespan

## Benefits of Companion Animals

The presence of a companion animal can have a positive effect on an individual's health status (Amiot, Bastian, & Martens, 2016; Friedman & Son, 2009). Relationships with animals may function as a form of social support that has health and well-being benefits (McNicholas & Collis, 2006). Therapeutic benefits of animals have been demonstrated in a variety of settings (McCardle, McCune, Griffin, Esposito, Freund, 2011) but findings related to the benefits of companion animals on owner well-being are inconsistent (Barker & Wolen, 2008; Headey, 2003; Herzog, 2011; Parslow, Jorm, Christensen, Rodgers, & Jacomb, 2005). Not all pets provide direct benefits such as companionship and exercise. And demands such as making time for

---

R. M. Bures (✉)
Eunice Kennedy Shriver National Institute of Child Health and Human Development (NICHD), National Institutes of Health, Bethesda, MD, USA

© The Author(s), under exclusive license to Springer Nature Switzerland AG 2021
R. Bures et al., *Well-Being Over the Life Course*,
SpringerBriefs in Well-Being and Quality of Life Research,
https://doi.org/10.1007/978-3-030-64085-9_3

an animal's needs or managing behavioral problems can create stressors for the pet owner (Serpell, 1996; Voith, 2009).

Having a pet serves as a resource that can buffer the impact of stressful events (Siegel, 1993). While both cat and dog owners often consider their pets to be family members (Arahori et al., 2017), the domestication history of the dog makes it a closer companion (Udell, Dorey, & Wynne, 2010). Benefits of companion animals may vary by the level and type of attachment. Individuals with high levels of attachment may consider their pet to be a family member, while others may see the pet as a working or practical companion. Companion animals develop attachment to humans as well, and this has been demonstrated for both dogs (Udell & Brubaker, 2016) and cats (Vitale, Behnke, & Udell, 2019).

For all their potential benefits, companion animals often have shorter life spans than humans (Triebenbacher, 2006). Aging takes its toll on pets much faster than it does on humans, and dealing with a sick or aging pet can be tough. Aging or ill animals may require additional care that is sometimes demanding (Christiansen, Kristensen, Sandøe, & Lassen, 2013). When a chronic disease or physical limitations manifest, the human caregiver usually adapts and makes the changes necessary to give the pet comfort. Often these adaptations become of part of the person's everyday life. The emotional and financial strains of caring for an ill or aging pet can manifest as caregiver stress, which in turn affects an individual's well-being.

## Family Caregiving and Stress

Since many pet owners consider their pets to be family members (see chapter "Integrating Pets into the Family Life Cycle" Bures, 2021), it makes sense to examine this form of human animal interaction as a family caregiving relationship. A family caregiving framework can be used as a tool to consider how companion animal illness and death may affect the well-being of their human caregivers. A substantial body of research exists on family caregiving (Pearlin, Mullan, Semple, & Skaff, 1990; Schulz & Sherwood, 2008; Schulz, Beach, Czaja, Martire, & Monin, 2020). Extending this concept to caring for pets can illuminate some of the challenges of pet ownership and attachment.

Caregiving can be a chronic stress experience (Schulz & Sherwood, 2008). It is associated with extended periods of physical and psychological strain and is characterized by unpredictability and uncontrollability. It can require high levels of attentiveness and potentially create secondary stress in family and work relationships. The level of chronic stress exposure from caregiving is dependent on the intensity of care provided and the level of suffering of the care recipient (Schulz et al., 2020).

Caregiver stress is not one size fits all. The stress of caregiving is a combination of circumstances, experiences, responses, and resources unique to each caregiver. As a result, it has different impacts on each caregivers' health and behavior (Pearlin et al., 1990). In their seminal work, Pearlin et al. outline what is known as the Stress Process Model of caregiving. This model describes caregiving as an adaptive developmental process comprising four domains: the context of the stress, the caregiving stressors, the mediators of stress, and the stress outcomes. Considering caregiver stress as a process shifts the attention to the interrelationships among the conditions leading to stress. For example, stress may be caused by interactions between the animal's health status, the costs of care, and the impact of caregiving on family and work relationships.

The stress of companion animal caregiving needs to be framed in its social context. Social ties may serve as a primary source of emotional support for individuals but, at the same time, social ties have the potential to be extremely stressful, such as close family relationships (Umberson & Karas Montez, 2010). To date there has been limited research on the impact of the relationship between the caregiver and care-receiver on caregiver well-being (Penning & Wu, 2015). Measurement of the impact of caregiving differs by age, gender, and type of caregiving as well as by the type of measure used.

There is little evidence from population-based studies that family caregivers, in general, have worse physical health than comparable non-caregiving groups (Roth, Fredman, & Haley, 2015). Yet there is substantial evidence that caregivers experience symptoms of emotional distress. It may be that stress is not generated by providing care as much as it is by observing a family member struggling with a serious medical condition (Monin & Schulz, 2009).

Like human caregiving, the impact of companion-animal care on caregiver well-being likely varies by marital status, gender, race/ethnicity, and socioeconomic status. Studies of gender differences in caregiving reveal that controlling for stressors and resources reduces the gender differences in physical health and depression to levels comparable to that observed in non-caregiving samples. These findings support stress-and-coping theories on gender differences in caregiving and are consistent with observations that men and women experience stress differently (Pinquart & Sörensen, 2006).

## Caregiver Burden

Advances in veterinary medicine mean that companion animals may live longer than in previous decades and that those with health issues may receive advanced care while still at home. With age, animals slow down. They may get aches and pains or develop chronic illnesses. Younger cats and dogs may also develop chronic conditions including kidney disease, epilepsy, or thyroid problems, which can make aging more difficult for the animal. Both aging and progressive illness can cause caregiver burden for an animal's human family. For individuals already burdened with caregiving for a human family member, an aging pet may create an additional burden (Connell, Janevic, Solway, & McLaughlin, 2007).

Companion animal illness may elevate caregiver burden for pet owners, but successful treatment of the condition may alleviate this burden. In a sample of dog owners, treatment of a dermatological condition that resulted in good skin disease control had no additional burden (Spitznagel et al., 2019). For dogs with epilepsy, treatment was associated with overall quality of life (Nettifee, Munana, & Griffith, 2017). Dogs with poorly controlled epilepsy or reactions to medications were reported to have lower quality of life.

To assess companion animal caregiver burden, Spitznagel, Jacobson, Cox, and Carlson (2017) used an adaptation of the Zarit Burden Interview (ZBI; see Zarit, Reever, & Bach-Peterson, 1980), replacing the words 'your relative/spouse' with 'your pet' in each item. Several items that were not relevant to the human–companion animal relationship were omitted, resulting in 18 items. Items in the adapted ZBI include feeling that it is painful to watch your pet age, feeling strained about your pet, experiencing a negative impact on social life, and having concerns about money. A score greater than 19 on the ZBI reflects "significant burden." In their matched sample, Spitznagel et al. reported average scores of 25.42 for caregivers of pets with a chronic or terminal disease and 13.96 for owners of healthy pets.

Understanding caregiver burden in the context of companion animals is important for understanding the owner's responsibilities and the veterinarian's roles and responsibilities for the care of seriously and terminally ill animals (Goldberg, 2017). Caregiver burden is a subjective and dynamic concept (Chou, 2000). Something considered a burden by one person may be acceptable to another. And as caregiving needs change, the perceived burden may change as well. But overall, for owners of companion animals with chronic or terminal illnesses, caregiver burden is linked to multiple negative psychosocial outcomes, including raised levels of stress, depressive and anxious symptoms, and lower quality of life (Spitznagel et al., 2017; Spitznagel, Jacobson, Cox, & Carlson, 2018).

## Companion Animal Illness and Loss

The life span of companion animals is relatively short, making the loss of an animal family member more common than the loss of a human family member (Cowles, 1985; Triebenbacher, 2006). For children, the loss of a pet may represent their first permanent loss; for adults, it may represent the loss of a beloved companion. Aging varies by species and breed, making it often difficult to characterize normal aging in companion animals (Szabó, Gee, & Miklósi, 2016).

Companion animal quality of life (QOL) is often a concern when there is an illness or advanced age. QOL extends beyond simple health to all dimensions of an animal's life (McMillan, 2003). Assessing QOL in companion animals is important for determining their well-being (McMillan, 2003; Mullan, 2015). Declining QOL is a common stressor for caregivers. There are numerous tools for assessing QOL in humans, but development and validation of tools to measure animal QOL has lagged (Belshaw, Asher, Harvey, & Dean, 2015; Mullan, 2015). Villalobos (1994) developed a Quality of Life Scale for terminally ill pets. The "HHHHHMM" Scale scores pets on a scale of 1 to 10 (ideal) on seven dimensions: hurt, hunger, hydration, hygiene, happiness, mobility, and more good days than bad. A score greater than 35 is considered acceptable.

One common theme related to the death of a pet is support from the veterinarian (Adams, Bonnett, & Meek, 2000; Ellwood, Simmonds, & Walker, 2001; Christiansen et al., 2013). Another is the need to deal with grief (Testoni et al., 2019). A study by Adams et al. (2000) found that 27% of participants experienced severe grief following the death of their cat or dog. Notable risk factors for grief included level of attachment, type of death, societal attitudes toward pet death, and veterinary support. These findings are consistent with results from an analysis of online responses to an article on the topic of losing a companion animal. Using qualitative thematic analysis, Laing and Maylea (2018, p. 221) identified four major themes: strength of the bond, anthropocentrically disenfranchised grief, anticipatory grief in the context of euthanasia, and the need for professional support.

Studying companion animal loss can be challenging because it may be difficult to share vulnerable and personal information (Furman, 2006). Individuals may be reluctant to share their grief for fear of ridicule (Gage & Holcomb, 1991). The loss of a pet can be disruptive to the family system (Triebenbacher, 2006; Walsh, 2009). The decision to proceed with euthanasia, which requires ending the life of another living being, can be a distinctive feature of the companion animal grief process (Reisbig, Hafen, Siqueira Drake, Girard, & Breunig, 2017). The decision related to the timing of euthanasia can be fraught with ethical and emotional strain, a topic that is often overlooked (Knesl et al., 2017).

Pet loss can be complicated and may result from things other than death of the animal (Walsh, 2009). For example, individuals with assistance animals may be separated due to retirement, reassignment, or death (Villalobos, 2019). Pet loss may also result from divorce (Fossati, 2020; Rook, 2014) and custody agreements based on child welfare. The loss of a pet impacts family functioning, and the associated grief may disrupt the lives of individual family members.

Heath care systems need to explicitly recognize the levels of grief and sadness experienced by some pet owners (Mohanti, 2017). In 2017, a 61-year old woman sought emergency treatment for heart-attack-like symptoms following the death of her dog (Maiti & Dhoble, 2017; Watson, 2017). She was diagnosed with broken heart syndrome, a temporary condition that is also known as stress-induced cardiomyopathy. The death of a companion animal can be like the loss of a family member (Carmack, 1985; Morris 2012) and can be a significant loss for individuals and families (Ellwood et al., 2001; Triebenbacher, 2006). The loss of a pet can be especially distressing if it was associated with a deceased spouse or regular social activities (McNicholas et al., 2005).

## Bereavement

Individuals who have lost a companion animal may experience denial, both of the animal's illness and the finality of its death, and feel anger that may be directed at the veterinarian (Cowles, 1985). An individual's level of attachment to their pet may affect how they deal with illness and loss of the animal (Serpell, 1996). In a sample of owners with euthanized pets, attachment to the pet was positively associated with feelings of sorrow and anger, and cancer diagnosis was negatively related to feelings of anger and guilt (Barnard-Nguyen, Breit, Anderson, & Nielsen, 2016). These experiences are consistent with the five stages of grief—denial, anger, depression, bargaining, acceptance—described by Kübler-Ross and Kessler (2005).

Yet grief does not follow prescribed stages. Doka and Davidson (2014, p. 2) describe individual differences that may affect the way grief manifests itself:

- the nature of the loss;
- the relationship and the attachment to the loss;
- circumstances surrounding the loss;
- the extent of, and response to, prior loss;
- the psychology and personality of the bereaved;
- personal variables such as health, lifestyle, and stress management; and a variety of social variables including age, gender, developmental level, social class, cultural and religious beliefs; and
- practices, family, and external and internal support.

Indeed, the main factors related to grief after the loss of a human relation (anger, guilt, grief, and intrusive thoughts) are often present after the loss of a pet (Uccheddu et al., 2019). Like human attachment, companion animal attachment is characterized by both attachment anxiety and avoidance (Zilcha-Mano, Mikulincer, & Shaver, 2011). Attachment anxiety is associated with closeness; avoidance is associated with emotional distance. Individuals with higher companion-animal attachment anxiety were found to grieve the death of a pet; those with higher avoidant attachment were relatively indifferent to the loss of their pet.

Using the Mourning Dog Questionnaire, a tool developed to assess owners' grief over the loss of a companion dog, the researchers found substantial variations in grief, likely due to individual differences in the way their grief is expressed (Uccheddu et al., 2019). Other results measuring grief and attachment demonstrate that dog owners tend to view human and animal relationships on the same continuum, not as separate entities. An understudied dimension of companion animal relationships is gender, as most respondents in studies of pet loss are female (Packman, Bussolari, Katz, & Carmack, 2016). Arguing that men grieve differently from women, not less, Packman et al. demonstrate that men have strong relationships with their dogs and experience deep grief at their loss.

Following the death of a companion animal, increased psychological support may help owners better cope with grief (Testoni, De Cataldo, Ronconi, & Zamperini, 2017) and professional support may be needed (Carmack, 1985; McCutcheon & Fleming, 2002). Effective communication from the veterinarian and veterinary team can help owners make conscious and informed end-of-life decisions and offer support (Testoni et al., 2017, 2019).

Support following the loss of a companion animal can be essential since the loss of a pet often goes unvalidated. The death of a companion animal may be accompanied by feelings of disenfranchised grief (Habarth et al., 2017; Packman, Bussolari, Katz, Carmack, & Field, 2014; Spain, O'Dwyer, & Moston, 2019; Testoni et al., 2017; Walsh, 2009). Friends, family, and the broader community may not recognize the loss of a pet as a "real loss" (Packman et al., 2014). Disenfranchised grief results from the experience of a loss that is either unacknowledged or considered insignificant. Consequently, the bereaved is unable to express their grief (Spain et al., 2019).

Dealing with disenfranchised grief may have an impact on an individual's psychosocial functioning. In this context, self-compassion training may have positive effects for bereaved pet owners (Bussolari, Habarth, Phillips, Katz, & Packman, 2019). Self-compassion may also moderate the relationships between grief severity and depression as well as between social constraints and depression. The social constraints related to grieving for the loss of a pet can have negative impacts on mental health and functional outcomes (Habarth et al., 2017).

## Continuing Bonds

As pets increasingly are considered family members, there is a parallel belief that pets have an afterlife (Davis, Irwin, Richardson, & O'Brien-Malone, 2003; Fidler, 2004; Testoni et al., 2017). Companion animals may be "granted a form of personhood that extends into the spiritual realm" (Magliocco, 2018, p. 62). The allegory of the Rainbow Bridge, an afterlife where companion animals are restored to their healthy states and await a reunion with their person, offers one example of a continuing bond, and serves as a tool for dealing with the loss of a pet:

> Just this side of heaven is a place called Rainbow Bridge.
>
> When an animal dies that has been especially close to someone here, that pet goes to Rainbow Bridge. There are meadows and hills for all of our special friends so they can run and play together. There is plenty of food, water and sunshine, and our friends are warm and comfortable. All the animals who had been ill and old are restored to health and vigor. Those who were hurt or maimed are made whole and strong again, just as we remember them in our dreams of days and times gone by.
>
> The animals are happy and content, except for one small thing; they each miss someone very special to them, who had to be left behind. They all run and play together, but the day comes when one suddenly stops and looks into the distance. His bright eyes are intent. His eager body quivers. Suddenly he begins to run from the group, flying over the green grass, his legs carrying him faster and faster.
>
> You have been spotted, and when you and your special friend finally meet, you cling together in joyous reunion, never to be parted again. The happy kisses rain upon your face; your hands again caress the beloved head, and you look once more into the trusting eyes of your pet, so long gone from your life but never absent from your heart.
>
> Then you cross Rainbow Bridge together.... (Author unknown, Brandes, 2009)

Both level of attachment to a companion animal and the length of the relationship are positively related to grief (Planchon, Templer, Stokes, & Keller, 2002). Coping with the loss of a companion animal can be complicated if the owner perceives that they have little social support (Rémillard, Meehan, Kelton, & Coe, 2017). Recommendations from a study of callers to a pet-loss support hotline included asking individuals to talk about their pet and exploring the strength of the caller's support network. Overcoming grief and finding ways to facilitate expressions of grief, such as memorials, may be necessary for posttraumatic growth (Spain et al., 2019).

Maintaining an emotional attachment, or continuing bonds, can facilitate grief reactions and mediate the impact of the loss of a companion animal on the bereaved owner (Packman, Carmack, & Ronen, 2012). These continuing bond expressions can include: recalling favorite memories, sensing an ongoing connection with the pet, thinking they heard or felt their pet; talking to their deceased pet; dreaming of the pet; holding on to collars or toys that belonged to their pet; creating memorials in tribute to their deceased pet; and having thoughts of being reunited with their pet (Habarth et al., 2017; Packman et al., 2012, p. 339).

Continuing bonds may help an individual resolve their grief, not by ending their relationship with their pet but by redefining it. Children often use continuing bonds to cope with the loss of a companion animal (Schmidt et al., 2020). This varies by the child's developmental stage and the level of attachment. For adults, the level of maintenance of continuing bonds for pets was similar to that for spouses (Packman, Field, Carmack, & Ronen, 2011). Maintaining a connection to a decreased pet through continuing bonds may be comforting, distressing, or both. Like grief, continuing bonds are unique to the individual and evolve over time (Packman et al., 2012).

## Conclusion

To understand the impact of the decline and death of companion animals on their owners and caregivers, researchers need to understand both the context of care and the emotional toll of caregiving. Human-animal interaction researchers increasingly draw on the family caregiving and bereavement literatures to better understand the consequences of the health and loss of a companion animal for individual well-being. Research on companion animal caregiving and loss may help to clarify conflicting findings related to the concept of a general "pet effect" on human health and well-being (Herzog, 2011).

One of the primary findings of human-animal interaction research has been that HAI increases well-being and reduces psychological distress, but more research is needed to clearly articulate the mechanisms of this relationship (Crossman, 2017). While the benefits of relationships with companion animals over their lives are considered worth the challenges that come with illness and death, the loss of a pet can cause extreme distress. The growing research on companion animal bereavement, particularly in association with euthanasia, is helping to illuminate this issue. Longitudinal research following the death of a companion animal may prove to be informative as well (Planchon et al., 2002).

In this chapter, the focus has been on companion animals whose owners have some form of attachment and maintain ownership. These relationships described cannot be expected with individuals who do not develop attachment and give up their animals. It should be noted that there is a separate literature on companion animal relinquishment, typically to animal shelters (see Arbe Montoya, Rand, Greer, Alberthsen, & Vankan, 2017; Lambert, Coe, Niel, Dewey, & Sargeant, 2019; Protopopova & Gunter, 2017).

A growing body of research on the consequences of companion-animal illness and loss for owner well-being builds on earlier companion-animal attachment research, as well as the broader literature on caregiving and grief. Advances have been made in the measurement of companion animal caregiver burden (Spitznagel et al., 2017) and grief following the loss of a pet (Uccheddu et al., 2019). Looking forward, researchers can explore the adaptation and testing of other health-related measures such as quality of life and general health. For example, self-rated health is frequently used as a general measure of human health and well-being (see Garbarski, 2016). Proxy reports of health have been shown to predict mortality as effectively as self-rated health (Ayalon & Covinsky, 2009), suggesting that a pet owner's report of an animal's health could be a reliable indicator. General measures of companion animal health should also be included in studies when possible.

There is also a need for better measurement of the owner's relationship with the companion animal in households with multiple animals, such as status within the companion-animal hierarchy. The inconsistency of instructions for individual animal selection in research shows a lack of standardization of studies of human–animal relationships more generally (Thompson, O'Dwyer, Bowen, & Smith, 2018). Researchers should explicitly consider the implications of companion animal selection methods (e.g., favorite pet) in an effort to match selection instructions with the specific research aims.

Future studies on the health and well-being effects of companion animal caregiving and loss should employ more rigorous research methodologies. Research findings to date have been consistent with the broader literature on grief, bereavement, and well-being, yet many studies have been based on convenience samples from veterinary clinics or online groups. There is a need for increased interdisciplinary collaboration and the inclusion of pet-related questions in longitudinal and population-based health surveys (McCune et al., 2014). While challenging, it would be useful to have study samples drawn from defined populations that would allow for well-being comparisons between companion animal owners and nonowners, as well as between caregivers and non-caregivers.

## References

Adams, C. L., Bonnett, B. N., & Meek, A. H. (2000). Predictors of owner response to companion animal death in 177 clients from 14 practices in Ontario. *Journal of the American Veterinary Medical Association, 217*(9), 1303–1309.

Amiot, C., Bastian, B., & Martens, P. (2016). People and companion animals: It takes two to tango. *BioScience, 66*(7), 552–560.

Arahori, M., Kuroshima, H., Hori, Y., Takagi, S., Chijiiwa, H., & Fujita, K. (2017). Owners' view of their pets' emotions, intellect, and mutual relationship: Cats and dogs compared. *Behavioural Processes, 141*, 316–321.

Arbe Montoya, A. I., Rand, J. S., Greer, R. M., Alberthsen, C., & Vankan, D. (2017). Relationship between sources of pet acquisition and euthanasia of cats and dogs in an animal shelter: A pilot study. *Australian Veterinary Journal, 95*(6), 194–200.

Ayalon, L., & Covinsky, K. E. (2009). Spouse-rated vs self-rated health as predictors of mortality. *Archives of Internal Medicine, 169*(22), 2156–2161.

Barker, S. B., & Wolen, A. R. (2008). The benefits of human–companion animal interaction: A review. *Journal of Veterinary Medical Education, 35*(4), 487–495.

Barnard-Nguyen, S., Breit, M., Anderson, K. A., & Nielsen, J. (2016). Pet loss and grief: Identifying at-risk pet owners during the euthanasia process. *Anthrozoös, 29*(3), 421–430.

Belshaw, Z., Asher, L., Harvey, N. D., & Dean, R. S. (2015). Quality of life assessment in domestic dogs: An evidence-based rapid review. *The Veterinary Journal, 206*(2), 203–212.

Brandes, S. (2009). The meaning of American pet cemetery gravestones. *Ethnology: An International Journal of Cultural and Social Anthropology, 48*(2), 99–118.

Bussolari, C., Habarth, J. M., Phillips, S., Katz, R., & Packman, W. (2019). Self-compassion, social constraints, and psychosocial outcomes in a pet bereavement sample. *OMEGA-Journal of Death and Dying,* 0030222818814050.

Carmack, B. J. (1985). The effects on family members and functioning after the death of a pet. *Marriage & Family Review, 8*(3–4), 149–161.

Chou, K. R. (2000). Caregiver burden: A concept analysis. *Journal of Pediatric Nursing, 15*(6), 398–407.

Christiansen, S. B., Kristensen, A. T., Sandøe, P., & Lassen, J. (2013). Looking after chronically ill dogs: Impacts on the caregiver's life. *Anthrozoös, 26*(4), 519–533.

Connell, C. M., Janevic, M. R., Solway, E., & McLaughlin, S. J. (2007). Are pets a source of support or added burden for married couples facing dementia? *Journal of Applied Gerontology, 26*(5), 472–485.

Cowles, K. V. (1985). The death of a pet: Human responses to the breaking of the bond. *Marriage & Family Review, 8*(3–4), 135–148.

Crossman, M. K. (2017). Effects of interactions with animals on human psychological distress. *Journal of Clinical Psychology, 73*(7), 761–784.

Davis, H., Irwin, P., Richardson, M., & O'Brien-Malone, A. (2003). When a pet dies: Religious issues, euthanasia and strategies for coping with bereavement. *Anthrozoös, 16*(1), 57–74.

Doka, K. J., & Davidson, J. D. (Eds.). (2014). *Living with grief: Who we are how we grieve.* New York: Routledge.

Ellwood, A., Simmonds, R., & Walker, J. (2001). Ask the animals, and they will teach you. *Family Medicine, 33*(7), 502–504.

Fidler, M. (2004). The question of animal immortality: Changing attitudes. *Anthrozoös, 17*(3), 259–266.

Fossati, P. (2020). Protecting Interests of Animals in Custody Disputes: Italian Caselaw Outpaces Italian and European Union Legislation. *Society & Animals, 1*(aop), 1–18.

Friedmann, E., & Son, H. (2009). The human–companion animal bond: How humans benefit. *Veterinary Clinics of North America: Small Animal Practice, 39*(2), 293–326.

Furman, R. (2006). Autoethnographic poems and narrative reflections: A qualitative study on the death of a companion animal. *Journal of Family Social Work, 9*(4), 23–38.

Gage, M. G., & Holcomb, R. (1991). Couples' perception of stressfulness of death of the family pet. *Family Relations, 40,* 103–105.

Garbarski, D. (2016). Research in and prospects for the measurement of health using self-rated health. *Public Opinion Quarterly, 80*(4), 977–997.

Goldberg, K. J. (2017). Exploring caregiver burden within a veterinary setting. *Veterinary Record, 181*(12), 318–319.

Habarth, J., Bussolari, C., Gomez, R., Carmack, B. J., Ronen, R., Field, N. P., & Packman, W. (2017). Continuing bonds and psychosocial functioning in a recently bereaved pet loss sample. *Anthrozoös, 30*(4), 651–670.

Headey, B. (2003). Pet ownership: good for health?. *Medical Journal of Australia, 179*(9), 460–461.

Herzog, H. (2011). The impact of pets on human health and psychological well-being: fact, fiction, or hypothesis? *Current Directions in Psychological Science, 20*(4), 236–239.

Knesl, O., Hart, B. L., Fine, A. H., Cooper, L., Patterson-Kane, E., Houlihan, K. E., & Anthony, R. (2017). Veterinarians and Humane endings: When is it the right time to euthanize a companion Animal? *Frontiers in Veterinary Science, 4*, 45.

Kübler-Ross, E., & Kessler, D. (2005). *On grief and grieving: Finding the meaning of grief through the five stages of loss.* New York: Simon and Schuster.

Laing, M., & Maylea, C. (2018). "They burn brightly, but only for a short time": The role of social workers in companion animal grief and loss. *Anthrozoös, 31*(2), 221–232.

Lambert, K., Coe, J., Niel, L., Dewey, C., & Sargeant, J. M. (2019). Companion-animal relinquishment: Exploration of the views expressed by primary stakeholders within published reviews and commentaries. *Society & Animals, 1*(aop), 1–22.

Magliocco, S. (2018). Beyond the rainbow bridge: Vernacular ontologies of animal afterlives. *Journal of Folklore Research, 55*(2), 39–68.

Maiti, A., Dhoble, A. (2017, October 19). Takotsubo cardiomyopathy. *New England Journal of Medicine: Images in Clinical Medicine, 377*, e24.

McCardle, P. D., McCune, S., Griffin, J. A., Esposito, L., & Freund, L. S. (Eds.). (2011). *Animals in our lives: Human-animal interaction in family, community, and therapeutic settings.* Baltimore, MD: Brookes.

McCune, S., Kruger, K. A., Griffin, J. A., Esposito, L., Freund, L. S., Hurley, K. J., & Bures, R. (2014). Evolution of research into the mutual benefits of human–animal interaction. *Animal Frontiers, 4*(3), 49–58.

McCutcheon, K. A., & Fleming, S. J. (2002). Grief resulting from euthanasia and natural death of companion animals. *OMEGA-Journal of Death and Dying, 44*(2), 169–188.

McMillan, F. D. (2003). Maximizing quality of life in Ill animals. *Journal of the American Animal Hospital Association, 39*(3), 227–235.

McNicholas, J., & Collis, G. M. (2006). Animals as social supports: Insights for understanding animal-assisted therapy. *Handbook on Animal-Assisted Therapy: Theoretical Foundations and Guidelines for Practice, 2*, 49–72.

McNicholas, J., Gilbey, A., Rennie, A., Ahmedzai, S., Dono, J. A., & Ormerod, E. (2005). Pet ownership and human health: A brief review of evidence and issues. *BMJ, 331*(7527), 1252–1254.

Mohanti, B. K. (2017). Grieving the Loss of a Pet Needs the Health System Recognition. *Journal of Social Work in End-of-Life & Palliative Care, 13*(4), 215–218.

Monin, J. K., & Schulz, R. (2009). Interpersonal effects of suffering in older adult caregiving relationships. *Psychology and Aging, 24*(3), 681.

Morris, P. (2012). Managing pet owners' guilt and grief in veterinary euthanasia encounters. *Journal of Contemporary Ethnography, 41*(3), 337–365.

Mullan, S. (2015). Assessment of quality of life in veterinary practice: Developing tools for companion animal carers and veterinarians. *Veterinary Medicine: Research and Reports, 6*, 203.

Nettifee, J. A., Munana, K. R., & Griffith, E. H. (2017). Evaluation of the impacts of epilepsy in dogs on their caregivers. *Journal of the American Animal Hospital Association, 53*(3), 143–149.

Packman, W., Bussolari, C., Katz, R., & Carmack, B. J. (2016). Continuing bonds research with animal companions: Implications for men grieving the loss of a dog. In *Men and their dogs* (pp. 303–320). Cham: Springer.

Packman, W., Bussolari, C., Katz, R., Carmack, B. J., & Field, N. P. (2014). Posttraumatic growth following the loss of a pet. *OMEGA-Journal of Death and Dying, 75*(4), 337–359.

Packman, W., Carmack, B. J., & Ronen, R. (2012). Therapeutic implications of continuing bonds expressions following the death of a pet. *OMEGA-Journal of Death and Dying, 64*(4), 335–356.

Packman, W., Field, N. P., Carmack, B. J., & Ronen, R. (2011). Continuing bonds and psychosocial adjustment in pet loss. *Journal of Loss and Trauma, 16*(4), 341–357.

Parslow, R. A., Jorm, A. F., Christensen, H., Rodgers, B., & Jacomb, P. (2005). Pet ownership and health in older adults: Findings from a survey of 2,551 community-based Australians aged 60–64. *Gerontology, 51*(1), 40–47.

Pearlin, L. I., Mullan, J. T., Semple, S. J., & Skaff, M. M. (1990). Caregiving and the stress process: An overview of concepts and their measures. *The Gerontologist, 30*(5), 583–594.

Penning, M. J., & Wu, Z. (2015). Caregiver stress and mental health: Impact of caregiving relationship and gender. *The Gerontologist, 56*(6), 1102–1113.

Pinquart, M., & Sörensen, S. (2006). Gender differences in caregiver stressors, social resources, and health: An updated meta-analysis. *The Journals of Gerontology Series B: Psychological Sciences and Social Sciences, 61*(1), P33–P45.

Planchon, L., Templer, D., Stokes, S., & Keller, J. (2002). Death of a companion cat or dog and human bereavement: Psychosocial variables. *Society & Animals, 10*(1), 93–105.

Protopopova, A., & Gunter, L. M. (2017). Adoption and relinquishment interventions at the animal shelter: A review. *Animal Welfare, 26*, 35–48.

Reisbig, A. M., Hafen, M., Jr., Siqueira Drake, A. A., Girard, D., & Breunig, Z. B. (2017). Companion animal death: A qualitative analysis of relationship quality, loss, and coping. *OMEGA-Journal of Death and Dying, 75*(2), 124–150.

Rémillard, L. W., Meehan, M. P., Kelton, D. F., & Coe, J. B. (2017). Exploring the grief experience among callers to a pet loss support hotline. *Anthrozoös, 30*(1), 149–161.

Rook, D. (2014). Who gets Charlie? The emergence of pet custody disputes in family law: Adapting theoretical tools from Child Law. *International Journal of Law, Policy and The Family, 28*(2), 177–193.

Roth, D. L., Fredman, L., & Haley, W. E. (2015). Informal caregiving and its impact on health: A reappraisal from population-based studies. *The Gerontologist, 55*(2), 309–319.

Schmidt, M., Naylor, P. E., Cohen, D., Gomez, R., Moses Jr, J. A., Rappoport, M., & Packman, W. (2020). Pet loss and continuing bonds in children and adolescents. *Death Studies, 44*(5), 278–284.

Schulz, R., Beach, S. R., Czaja, S. J., Martire, L. M., & Monin, J. K. (2020). Family caregiving for older adults. *Annual Review of Psychology, 71*, 635–659.

Schulz, R., & Sherwood, P. R. (2008). Physical and mental health effects of family caregiving. *Journal of Social Work Education, 44*(sup3), 105–113.

Serpell, J. A. (1996). Evidence for an association between pet behavior and owner attachment levels. *Applied Animal Behaviour Science, 47*(1–2), 49–60.

Siegel, J. M. (1993). Companion animals: In sickness and in health. *Journal of Social Issues, 49*(1), 157–167.

Spain, B., O'Dwyer, L., & Moston, S. (2019). Pet Loss: Understanding Disenfranchised Grief, Memorial Use, and Posttraumatic Growth. *Anthrozoös, 32*(4), 555–568.

Spitznagel, M. B., Jacobson, D. M., Cox, M. D., & Carlson, M. D. (2017). Caregiver burden in owners of a sick companion animal: A cross-sectional observational study. *Veterinary Record, vetrec-2017, 181*(12), 321.

Spitznagel, M. B., Jacobson, D. M., Cox, M. D., & Carlson, M. D. (2018). Predicting caregiver burden in general veterinary clients: Contribution of companion animal clinical signs and problem behaviors. *The Veterinary Journal, 236*, 23–30.

Spitznagel, M. B., Solc, M., Chapman, K. R., Updegraff, J., Albers, A. L., & Carlson, M. D. (2019). Caregiver burden in the veterinary dermatology client: Comparison to healthy controls and relationship to quality of life. *Veterinary Dermatology, 30*(1), 3–e2.

Szabó, D., Gee, N. R., & Miklósi, Á. (2016). Natural or pathologic? Discrepancies in the study of behavioral and cognitive signs in aging family dogs. *Journal of Veterinary Behavior, 11*, 86–98.

Testoni, I., De Cataldo, L., Ronconi, L., Colombo, E. S., Stefanini, C., Dal Zotto, B., & Zamperini, A. (2019). Pet grief: Tools to assess owners' bereavement and veterinary communication skills. *Animals, 9*(2), 67.

Testoni, I., De Cataldo, L., Ronconi, L., & Zamperini, A. (2017). Pet loss and representations of death, attachment, depression, and euthanasia. *Anthrozoös, 30*(1), 135–148.

Thompson, K., O'Dwyer, L., Bowen, H., & Smith, B. (2018). One dog, but which dog? How researchers guide participants to select dogs in surveys of human–dog relationships. *Anthrozoös, 31*(2), 195–210.

Triebenbacher, S. L. (2006). The companion animal within the family system: The manner in which animals enhance life within the home. In *Handbook on animal-assisted therapy* (pp. 357–374). San Diego: Academic Press.

Uccheddu, S., De Cataldo, L., Albertini, M., Coren, S., Da Graça Pereira, G., Haverbeke, A., ... Testoni, I. (2019). Pet humanisation and related grief: Development and validation of a structured questionnaire instrument to evaluate grief in people who have lost a companion dog. *Animals, 9*(11), 933.

Udell, M. A., & Brubaker, L. (2016). Are dogs social generalists? Canine social cognition, attachment, and the dog-human bond. *Current Directions in Psychological Science, 25*(5), 327–333.

Udell, M. A., Dorey, N. R., & Wynne, C. D. (2010). What did domestication do to dogs? A new account of dogs' sensitivity to human actions. *Biological Reviews, 85*(2), 327–345.

Umberson, D., & Karas Montez, J. (2010). Social relationships and health: A flashpoint for health policy. *Journal of Health and Social Behavior, 51*(1_suppl), S54–S66.

Villalobos, A. (1994). *Quality of Life Scale Helps Make Final Call, VPN.* Retrieved from https://pawspice.com/quality-of-life-scale.html.

Villalobos, A. E. (2019). Supporting people with disabilities endure the loss of their assistance animals at end of service or at end of life: An uplifting RETHINK for all involved. *Frontiers in Veterinary Science, 6,* 309.

Vitale, K. R., Behnke, A. C., & Udell, M. A. (2019). Attachment bonds between domestic cats and humans. *Current Biology, 29*(18), R864–R865.

Voith, V. L. (2009). The impact of companion animal problems on society and the role of veterinarians. *Veterinary Clinics of North America: Small Animal Practice, 39*(2), 327–345.

Walsh, F. (2009). Human-Animal bonds II: The role of pets in family systems and family therapy. *Family Process, 48*(4), 481–499.

Watson, R. (2017, October 23). *Broken heart syndrome redux: Woman suffers after dog's death* [Blog Post]. Retrieved from https://www.psychologytoday.com/us/blog/love-and-gratitude/201710/broken-heart-syndrome-redux-woman-suffers-after-dog-s-death.

Zarit, S. H., Reever, K. E., & Bach-Peterson, J. (1980). Relatives of the impaired elderly: Correlates of feelings of burden. *The Gerontologist, 20*(6), 649–655.

Zilcha-Mano, S., Mikulincer, M., & Shaver, P. R. (2011). An attachment perspective on human-pet relationships: Conceptualization and assessment of pet attachment orientations. *Journal of Research in Personality, 45*(4), 345–357.


**Regina M. Bures, Ph.D.** is a Senior Program Director in the Population Dynamics Branch at the *Eunice Kennedy Shriver* National Institute of Child Health and Human Development (NICHD) at the National Institutes of Health. At NICHD, Dr. Bures manages a diverse scientific portfolio in demography and population health. She has been an active contributor to the NICHD-Waltham partnership. Dr. Bures received her Ph.D. in Sociology, with a specialization in Demography, from Brown University and completed a postdoctoral fellowship at the University of Chicago. Dr. Bures has received numerous grants and awards, including research funding from the National Science Foundation and the National Institute of Aging. Her research interests include human-animal interaction, child and family health across the life course, data science, and research methods. She currently lives outside Washington, DC, with her husband, cats, dogs, and sheep.

# Health over the Life Course and Human-Animal Interaction

**Regina M. Bures, Layla Esposito, and James A. Griffin**

**Abstract** Research on the relationship between human animal interaction (HAI) and health and well-being over the life course typically focuses on specific age groups. This is particularly the case in the United States where HAI measures have not historically been included in longitudinal studies. We present a brief overview of the role of companion animals in healthy development and aging over the life course and evidence of how HAI may affect those processes. Limitations of research on HAI and health to date are discussed with a focus on the need to include measures of pet ownership and attachment in population representative samples to facilitate secondary analysis. Several population-representative data resources that can be used to study HAI across the life course in the United States are described: the Panel Study of Income Dynamics Child Development Supplement, the Early Childhood Longitudinal Study—Kindergarten Cohort, the General Social Survey, and the Health and Retirement Study. Opportunities for researchers to contribute to the growing multidisciplinary field of HAI research are discussed.

**Keywords** Animal assisted therapy · Pet therapy · Stress reduction · Pets · Companion animals · Life course · Family life cycle · Child development · Caregiving · Stress · Aging · Health · Well-being · Bereavement · Human-animal interaction · Human-animal bond · Lifespan

Health and well-being are fundamental issues across the life course. While the dimensions of what constitutes health and well-being changes as individuals age, human-animal interaction (HAI) also varies across the life course. The range of interactions between individuals and companion animals over the life course and the impact

---

R. M. Bures (✉) · L. Esposito · J. A. Griffin
Eunice Kennedy Shriver National Institute of Child Health and Human Development (NICHD), National Institutes of Health, Bethesda, MD, USA

L. Esposito
e-mail: espositl@mail.nih.gov

J. A. Griffin
e-mail: james.griffin@nih.gov

of those interactions on outcomes ranging from child development to successful aging are increasingly of interest to HAI researchers. The role of interaction with a companion animal in an individual's life and how they are affected by that interaction varies across the course of human development. For example, the way a toddler interacts with and benefits from a pet is likely quite different than how a young adult or an elderly person might. This is a distinguishing characteristic of HAI research: the focus shifts from the individual to the relationship between the individual and the animal (Amiot & Bastian, 2015), particularly when interactions involve companion animals such as dogs or cats.

## Human-Animal Interaction and Health

Healthy companion animals may contribute to better human health (Rock, Mykhalovskiy, & Schlich, 2007). There are a number of reasons for this potential relationship. Human-animal interaction is often associated with positive emotional development in childhood, lower BMI and increased physical activity among adults, and the retention of mobility and independence among the elderly (see review by Headey & Grabka, 2011). While companion animal support cannot be viewed as a replacement for human interactions, pets, by not being humans, may offer more stable relationships and with no concerns about commitment (McNicholas et al., 2005).

## Child Health and Well-Being

Researchers increasingly focus on the relationships between role of pets in child development, health, and well-being. Interactions with a family pet or therapeutic animal interventions can influence children's social, emotional, cognitive and health outcomes (e.g., Esposito, McCune, Griffin, & Maholmes, 2011; McCardle, McCune, Griffin, Esposito, & Freund, 2010; McCardle, McCune, Griffin, & Maholmes, 2010). For example, animals can influence the development of social competence by strengthening empathy, serving as a catalyst for social interaction, improving relationships, and providing emotional support. The presence of animals in classrooms can motivate children to learn and improve a wide range of developmental skills (McCardle, McCune, Griffin, Esposito et al., 2010). A companion animal may stimulate a young child's curiosity and learning, in addition to providing emotional support to the child (Melson, 2003). Animal-assisted activities in the classroom have been shown to increase social skills and decrease problem behaviors (O'Haire, McKenzie, McCune, & Slaughter, 2013).

Research has demonstrated an association between human-animal interaction and physiological and health outcomes (e.g., Esposito et al., 2011). For example, dog ownership is associated with reduced obesity in childhood. Researchers have found that children in families who own dogs were less likely to be overweight or obese, compared to families without a dog (Timperio, Salmon, Chu, & Andrianopoulos, 2008).

Human-animal interaction is used in a variety of settings to support children with health, behavioral or emotional problems. Animals or animal puppets and toys may be used to facilitate communication in therapeutic pediatric settings (Goddard & Gilmer, 2015; Melson & Fine, 2015). Animals can provide emotional support to children, especially for children experiencing difficult or stressful situations (Nagengast, Baun, Megel, & Liebowitz, 1997). Researchers have found that positive physical and psychological outcomes are associated with the social support that animals can provide (Allen, 1997; Garrity & Stallones, 1998; Redefer & Goodman, 1989).

The positive impact of animals on child development extends beyond interactions with companion animals. Research has also demonstrated the benefits of horseback riding with respect to enhancing physical health (Clutterbuck, Auld, & Johnston, 2019), as well as positive outcomes associated with child development. For example, one study found that for children rated as having low social competence, an equine facilitated learning program improved social competence and behavior (Pendry, Carr, Smith, & Roeter, 2014) and had lower afternoon cortisol levels compared to children on the waitlist (Pendry, Smith, & Roeter, 2014). For horseback riding, one hypothesized mechanism of change appears to be the growth of self through learning to move, connect, and adapt (Ohtani et al., 2017). Therapies such as horseback riding can be applied to other life contexts to promote development and growth (Martin, Graham, Taylor, & Levack, 2018).

## Adult Health and Well-Being and HAI

In adults, pet ownership is commonly associated with better health outcomes. This relationship depends on the type of pet: Cat and dog owners are more likely to engage in health behaviors such as regular exercise (Utz, 2014). Pet ownership, particularly dog ownership, may be associated with decreased risk of developing cardiovascular disease (Levine et al., 2013). One mechanism for some of the benefits of dog ownership may be the increased physical activity. Dog walking is associated with increased physical activity (Reeves, Rafferty, Miller, & Lyon-Callo, 2011), as well as lower BMI, and lower levels of diabetes, hypertension, and depression (Lentino, Visek, McDonnell, & DiPietro, 2012), and lower risk of death (Kramer, Mehmood, & Suen, 2019). Dog walking is also associated with increased social interactions (McNichols & Collis, 2000; Wood et al., 2015).

Examining human-dog interactions, Odendaal and Meintjes (2003) suggest that the benefits of human-companion animal interaction are probably based on a form of reciprocity, where both humans and dogs benefit from positive interactions. There is evidence that interaction with animals is associated with stress reduction (Baun, Oetting, & Bergstrom, 1991; Viau et al., 2010) and improved physiological responses, including cortisol and epinephrine production, blood pressure, and heart rate variability (i.e., Allen, Shykoff, & Izzo, 2001; Anderson, Reid, & Jennings, 1992; Wilson, 1987).

Having a pet may also encourage social contact and interaction in a community (Wood, Giles-Corti, & Bulsaras, 2005). Pet ownership alone may not be associated with health status, but pet attachment has been found to be associated with decreased depression among the elderly (Garrity, Stallones, Marx, & Johnson, 1989). In hospital settings, visiting family pets were associated with increased communication between family members, providers, and patients that resulted in compassion, connection, and positive responses (Yamasaki, 2018).

Yet the evidence on the impact of pets on human health and well-being to date has been inconsistent and inconclusive (Herzog, 2011). Healthiest adults, defined as those having made the fewest doctor visits, were long-term pet owners (Headey & Gradka 2007). In the Chinese context, dogs have been associated with better health outcomes (Headey, Na, & Zheng, 2008). At older ages, Parslow, Jorm, Christensen, Rodgers, and Jacomb (2005) found no evidence of health benefits of pet ownership. McColgan and Schofield (2007) suggest that dogs, in particular, can improve and help the emotional and physical well-being of older people.

It is likely that pet ownership has both positive (Headey, 2003) and negative effects on adult health, with analyses resulting in statistically significant associations depending on factors including the observed outcome (Hodgson et al., 2015), the composition of the analytic sample, and covariates utilized in the analysis (Griffin, Hurley, & McCune, 2020; Mueller, Gee, & Bures, 2018). Thus, it is very important to examine the health benefits of companion, therapy and service animals, including the mechanisms through which health gains are realized (Serpell, McCune, Gee, & Griffin, 2017), and to acknowledge the strengths and limitations of the corpus of research used as the basis for statements by, for example, the American Heart Association (Levine et al., 2013) and the Mayo Clinic (Creagan, Bauer, Thomley, & Borg, 2015).

## Research Gaps

The field of HAI presents multiple research opportunities. Despite the research to date, there remain significant gaps in our knowledge of the social and health consequences of human-animal interaction. Many HAI studies have been based on small samples limited to pet owners or those interacting with animals. Some larger surveys in Europe and Australia (e.g. the Avon Longitudinal Study of Parents and Children, the German Socioeconomic Panel, and the Australian National Social Science Survey) have incorporated HAI measures but large surveys in the United States have historically not included questions related to human-animal interaction. When HAI questions have been included in U.S. studies, they are often related to a single topic such as pet ownership or dog walking behavior. These types of questions have been included in a number of studies including the Michigan Behavioral Risk Factor Survey and the Health, Aging and Body Composition Study, and NHANES III.

What is missing from these large U.S. surveys are the consistent inclusion of measures of both pet ownership and human-animal attachment. Research has demonstrated that well-being is affected by relationships and levels of attachment over the life course (Sable, 1995; Stallones, Marx, Garrity, & Johnson, 1990). To understand the full impact of pets and human-animal interaction on health and well-being, surveys need to include measures of type of pet as well as attachment (Hawkins & Williams, 2017; Zasloff, 1996). In addition, many HAI studies are cross-sectional and based on small or convenience samples (Friedman & Gee, 2018). As the field grows, there remains a pressing need for data from population representative samples that will increase the generalizability of results and permit researchers to examine selection into pet ownership as well as pet-related outcomes.

In 2008, NICHD and the WALTHAM® Centre for Pet Nutrition, a division of Mars, Inc., entered into a public-private partnership to study human-animal interaction. This partnership seeks to encourage HAI research on child health and development as well as HAI research on health and development across the entire life course. Given the changing roles that pets play throughout people's lives and the potential connection between HAI and well-being over the life course, the partnership has emphasized the need for both additional research and better HAI data (see McCune, Kruger, Griffin, Esposito, Freund, Hurley, & Bures, 2014). One of the accomplishments of this partnership has been to support the development of a series of brief HAI questions and supporting the inclusion of these questions in several population representative studies in the US. The attachment questions were based on a subset of questions from the CENSHARE Pet Attachment Survey (see Holcomb, Williams, & Richards, 1985). The next section provides a brief overview of each of these new data resources for population representative studies of HAI in the United States. These include:

- Panel Study of Income Dynamics, Child Development Supplement (PSID CDS), 2014 & 2019
- Early Childhood Longitudinal Study—Kindergarten Cohort 2011 (ECLS-K:2011)
- General Social Survey (GSS), 2018
- Health and Retirement Study (HRS), 2012 HAI Module.

Data from all of these studies is publicly accessible via the respective study website.

## Panel Study of Income Dynamics, Child Development Supplement (PSID CDS)

The Panel Study of Income Dynamics (PSID) is a longitudinal, nationally representative household survey that began in 1968. The original sample comprised over 18,000 individuals living in 5,000 families in the United States. The PSID Child Development Supplement (CDS) is a supplemental study to the main study. The first CDS study collected data on a sample of children from PSID families who were 0 to 12 years old in 1997, and followed those children over three waves, ending in 2007–2008. The CDS-2014 includes all eligible children in PSID households born since 1997. For additional information on the PSID CDS see https://psidonline.isr.umich.edu/Studies.aspx.

The CDS-2014 provided an opportunity to incorporate pet and HAI measures into a large sample of American children for the first time. The CDS-2014 sample is a nationally representative sample of approximately 6,800 American children aged 0 to 17 years. The data were collected through interviews with primary caregivers (PCGs) and with older children themselves (ages 8–17 years). The CDS 2014 also includes a diary study of children's time use.

Primary caregivers (PCGs) are parents/guardians, typically mothers, who co-reside with CDS children and answer questions about each CDS child and about themselves and the household environment. The PCGs were asked about the number and types of family pets as well as the PCG's interaction with and attitudes about their pets. The pet-related items for PCGs included number and type of current pets, whether the family had a pet 5 years ago, reasons for not owning a pet, and three questions related to pet attachment.

Older children were asked questions about the characteristics of their pets and their interactions with family pets, including whether they had a pet as well as a favorite pet, type of pet, and six questions about pet attachment. For a detailed description of the CDS-2014 attachment measures see Bures, Mueller, and Gee (2019). The questions are repeated in the CDS-2019.

The CDS-2014 pet and attachment questions represent the inclusion of the first detailed measures of pet ownership and attachment in a population representative study of children in the United States. The HAI-related measures are part of a larger set of contextual factors describing families' resources and social environments and children's well-being. For example, other measures already included in the CDS survey will track changes in families' housing and neighborhoods, social assistance program use, employment, parental and family relationships, and social support.

The addition of these questions to the CDS-2014 provided baseline measures of pet ownership and attachment as well as detailed measures of child development that can be revisited in future waves of data collection. These data are publicly available via the PSID Data Center (https://simba.isr.umich.edu/data/data.aspx) and can be used by researchers interested in a wide variety of questions on child development, including the impact of children's HAI experiences on developmental outcomes.

## Early Childhood Longitudinal Study—Kindergarten Cohort 2011 (ECLS-K:2011)

The Early Childhood Longitudinal Study—Kindergarten Cohort 2011 (ECLS-K:2011) is a study sponsored by the National Center for Education Statistics (NCES), US Department of Education. The ECLS-K:2011 followed a cohort of children from their kindergarten year (the 2010–2011 school year) through the 2015–2016 school year, when most of the children were in the fifth grade (see https://nces.ed.gov/ecls/kindergarten2011.asp for study resources as well as a link to the public use data files). During the 2010–2011 school year both fall and spring data collections were conducted. The original ECLS-K:2011 sample is comprised of approximately 18,170 kindergartners from an estimated 1,310 schools and their parents, teachers, school administrators, and before- and after-school care providers participated in the study (see Tourangeau et al., 2018).

The children in the ECLS-K:2011 comprise a nationally representative sample selected from both public and private schools attending both full-day and part-day kindergarten in 2010–2011. Data are linked to child, family and school data collected from the time the children entered Kindergarten onward. While the ECLS-K refers to each round of data collection by the grade the children were expected to be in, all originally sampled children were included in the follow-up data collection regardless of their grade level. The ECLS-K:2011 included pet and attachment questions in the Fourth Grade Child Questionnaire and a therapy dog question in both the Fourth and Fifth Grade Special Education Teacher Questionnaire—Child Level (see https://nces.ed.gov/ecls/instruments2011.asp).

Children were asked whether they have a family pet or ever had one. Children who have at least one pet were asked: how old they were when they got their first pet; the number and kind(s) of pet they have; whether they have a favorite pet (and which one it is). The children with pets were also asked questions assessing their attachment to their pet, such as time spent playing with the pet, proximity of the pet when doing things like homework or watching TV, seeking the pet for comfort, and whether the pet is considered a member of the family.

Special education teacher questionnaires at the child level asked about animal assisted therapy (AAT). Specifically, the teachers were asked: "During this school year, has this child had the assistance of a service animal while at school? A service animal is any guide dog, signal dog, or other dog individually trained to provide assistance to an individual with a disability. Service animals can be used full time or in-school only as part of a program such as animal assisted therapy (AAT)."

The inclusion of these questions in the ECLS-K:2011 provides opportunities for researchers to explore the ways that pet ownership and attachment may influence children's school performance, school engagement, social relationships, health, and well-being. Because this is a nationally representative sample, the data from the inclusion of these questions may also help researchers better understand whether and HAI may serve as a protective buffer for children experiencing stressful home situations or social, emotional, or learning challenges (Gee, Griffin, & McCardle, 2017).

## General Social Survey (GSS)

The General Social Survey (GSS) is a bi-annual, cross-sectional population representative household-based survey of adults aged 18 and older which is conducted by NORC at the University of Chicago (see https://gss.norc.org/). Since 1972, the GSS has collected data for the purpose of monitoring changes in both social characteristics and attitudes in the United States. For more information about the GSS, including data access, see https://gss.norc.org/.

The NICHD-WALTHAM partnership supported the addition of a module adding survey questions on pet ownership and human-animal interaction (HAI) to the 2018 GSS. This module was asked to half of the GSS sample ($n = 1,250$). The added questions were derived from those included in the 2014 Panel Study of Income Dynamics (PSID) Child Development Supplement (CDS) and the Health and Retirement Study (HRS) 2012 module 9, which had been based on the CENSHARE Pet Attachment Survey (Holcomb et al., 1985).

Pet ownership and attachment questions were asked, including the number of pets does the family has; why the family doesn't have a pet; whether the family had a pet 5 years ago; type(s) of pet; and 3 attachment questions. The attachment questions were also asked of respondents how reported having a pet 4 years ago.

Data collected by the GSS include an array of demographic, social, and attitude variables. The inclusion of pet ownership and attachment questions in the GSS provides the opportunity for researchers to explore the associations between having a pet and human-animal interaction across a wide range of social and demographic variables in a U.S.-based population representative survey of adults.

## Health and Retirement Study (HRS)

Health and Retirement Study (HRS) is an ongoing biennial longitudinal cohort study of approximately 20,000 Americans aged 50 and older and, if married, their spouses, regardless of the spouse's age. HRS Core respondents are re-interviewed at two-year intervals and the sample has been replenished multiple times since the study originated in 1992. The HRS contains detailed information on family structure and composition, health, and labor force participation.

The HRS has included questions on pets in two waves data collection: the 2011 Internet Survey and an experimental module in the 2012 biannual survey. A 2011 Internet Survey included a section on Pets. Questions were asked about pet-related spending as well as currently or ever had a pet(s), type of pet, major reason for getting pet, who cares for pet, time spent walking dog (dog owner's), and pet's most endearing trait.

The HRS 2012 included an experimental module on HAI (Module 9). For HRS modules, participants are randomly assigned to one experimental module per wave; of the 20,554 total respondents in Wave 12, a random subsample of 2,037 were assigned to the HAI module. This module included questions about current and former pets, reasons for not having a pet, and responsibility for pet. Six questions on attachment to both current and, if no current, former pets were asked. These were based on the CENSHARE Pet Attachment Questionnaire (Anderson, 2006; Holcomb et al., 1985; Garrity et al., 1989). In addition, multiple questions were asked about dog walking. For a detailed overview of the HAI data in the 2012 HRS see Mueller et al. (2018).

The HRS 2012 was the first nationally representative survey in the United States to include measures of HAI in this detail. The inclusion of the HAI module in the HRS 2012 made a significant contribution to HAI research in two ways: by contributing to the development of tools and methods to measure HAI and, as a result, providing an opportunity for researchers to use secondary analysis to contribute to our knowledge of the ways that HAI contributes to individual wellbeing. These data provide researchers with the opportunity to better understand the relationship between pet ownership and attachment and the social, physical and mental well-being of the HRS study respondents. The Core HRS contains a wide array of measures that could be used in analyses with the HAI measures including demographics, family structure, employment status, ADLs, physical impairment, cognition, depression, social support, numbers of chronic conditions and healthcare utilization. Data are available through the HRS website (https://hrs.isr.umich.edu/data-products).

## Conclusion

Given the importance of companion animals in the lives of individuals, children, and families, there is an ongoing effort to develop a strong scientific base to help researchers more fully understand the ways that HAI can contribute to better health outcomes (Esposito, McCardle, Maholmes, McCune, & Griffin, 2010). The inclusion of measures of pet ownership and attachment in ongoing studies is one step toward developing this base. Longitudinal and repeated measures will move the field forward by facilitating research on the mechanisms that explain why and under what circumstances interactions with animals promote positive child development as well as positive physical health outcomes and the promotion of healthy lifestyles across the life course. Potential research questions to be explored at the population-level include: the impact of having and interacting with a pet on the social, emotional and cognitive abilities of children, adults, and older individuals; the extent to which pets serve as a buffer in family and social dynamics; and the conditions under which dog ownership promotes walking activity across the life course.

This brief overview of some of the key issues in research on human-animal interaction, health, and well-being over the life course sets the stage for the following chapters. As human-animal interaction research shifts the focus of research from the individual to the relationship and interaction between the individual and the animal, particularly when that interaction involves pets such as dogs or cats, we will gain a better understanding of the underlying mechanisms through which our companion animals may influence our health and well-being.

# References

Allen, D. (1997). Effects of dogs on human health. *Journal of the American Veterinary Medical Association, 210,* 1136–1139.

Allen, K., Shykoff, B., & Izzo, J. (2001). Pet Ownership, but not ace inhibitor therapy blunts home blood pressure responses to mental stress. *Hypertension, 38,* 815–820.

Amiot, C. E., & Bastian, B. (2015). Toward a psychology of human–animal relations. *Psychological Bulletin, 141*(1), 6.

Anderson, D. C. (Ed.). (2006). *Assessing the human-animal bond: A compendium of actual measures.* West Lafayette: Purdue University Press.

Anderson, W., Reid, C., & Jennings, L. (1992). Pet ownership and risk factors for cardiovascular disease. *Medical Journal of Australia, 157,* 298–301.

Baun, M., Oetting, K., & Bergstrom, N. (1991). Health benefits of companion animals in relation to the physiologic indices of relaxation. *Holistic Nursing Practice, 15,* 16–23.

Bures, R. M., Mueller, M. K., & Gee, N. R. (2019). Measuring human-animal attachment in a large US survey: Two brief measures for children and their primary caregivers. *Frontiers in Public Health, 7,* 107.

Clutterbuck, G., Auld, M., & Johnston, L. (2019). Active exercise interventions improve gross motor function of ambulant/semi-ambulant children with cerebral palsy: A systematic review. *Disability and Rehabilitation, 41*(10), 1131–1151.

Creagan, E. T., Bauer, B. A., Thomley, B.S., Borg, J. M. (2015). Animal-assisted therapy at Mayo Clinic: The time is now. *Complementary Therapies in Clinical Practice, 21*(2), 101–104. https://doi.org/10.1016/j.ctcp.2015.03.002.

Esposito, L. E., McCardle, P., Maholmes, V., McCune, S., & Griffin, J. A. (2010). Introduction. In P. McCardle, M. McCune, J. A., Griffin, L., Esposito, & L. Freund (Eds.), *Animals in our lives: Human-animal interaction in family, community, & therapeutic settings* (pp. 1–5). Baltimore: Brookes.

Esposito, L., McCune, S., Griffin, J., & Maholmes, V. (2011). Directions in human-animal interaction research: child development, health, and therapeutic interventions. *Child Development Perspectives, 0,* 1–7.

Friedmann, E., & Gee, N. R. (2018). Critical review of research methods used to consider the impact of human–animal interaction on older adults' health. *The Gerontologist, 59*(5), 964–972.

Garrity, T. F., & Stallones, L. (1998). Effects of pet contact on human well-being: Review of recent research. In C. C. Wilson & D. C. Turner (Eds.), *Companion animals in human health* (pp. 3–23). London: Sage.

Garrity, T. F., Stallones, L. F., Marx, M. B., & Johnson, T. P. (1989). Pet ownership and attachment as supportive factors in the health of the elderly. *Anthrozoös, 3*(1), 35–44.

Gee, NR., Griffin, J. A., & McCardle, P. M. (2017). Human-Animal Interaction Research in School Settings: Current Knowledge and Future Directions. *AERA Open, 3*(3), 1–9. https://doi.org/10.1177%2F2332858417724346.

Goddard, A. T., & Gilmer, M. J. (2015). The role and impact of animals with pediatric patients. *Pediatric Nursing, 41*(2), 65.

Griffin, J. A., Hurley, K., & McCune, S. (2020). Human-Animal Interaction research: Progress and possibilities. *Frontiers in Psychology.* https://doi.org/10.3389/fpsyg.2019.02803.

Hawkins, R., & Williams, J. (2017). Childhood attachment to pets: Associations between pet attachment, attitudes to animals, compassion, and humane behaviour. *International Journal of Environmental Research and Public Health, 14*(5), 490.

Headey, B. (2003). Pet ownership: Good for health? *Medical Journal of Australia, 179*(9), 460–461.

Headey, B., & Grabka, M. M. (2007). Pets and human health in Germany and Australia: National longitudinal results. *Social Indicators Research, 80*(2), 297–311.

Headey, B., & Grabka, M. (2011). Health correlates of pet ownership from national surveys. In P. McCardle, S. McCune, J. A. Griffin, & V. Maholmes (Eds.), *How animals affect us: Examining the influence of human–animal interaction on child development and human health* (pp. 153–162). Washington, DC: American Psychological Association.

Headey, B., Na, F., & Zheng, R. (2008). Pet dogs benefit owners' health: A 'natural experiment' in China. *Social Indicators Research, 87*(3), 481–493.

Herzog, H. (2011). The impact of pets on human health and psychological well-being: Fact, fiction, or hypothesis? *Current Directions in Psychological Science, 20*(4), 236–239.

Hodgson, K., Barton, L., Darling, M., Antao, V., Kim, F. A., & Monavvari, A. (2015). Pets' impact on your patients' health: Leveraging benefits and mitigating risk. *The Journal of the American Board of Family Medicine, 28*(4), 526–534.

Holcomb, R., Williams, R. C., & Richards, P.S. (1985). The elements of attachment: Relationship maintenance and intimacy. *Journal of the Delta Society, 2*(1), 28–34.

Kramer, C. K., Mehmood, S., & Suen, R. S. (2019). Dog ownership and survival: a systematic review and meta-analysis. *Circulation: Cardiovascular Quality and Outcomes, 12*(10), e005554.

Lentino, C., Visek, A. J., McDonnell, K., & DiPietro, L. (2012). Dog walking is associated with a favorable risk profile independent of a moderate to high volume of physical activity. *Journal of Physical Activity and Health, 9*(3), 414–420.

Levine, G. N., Allen, K., Braun, L. T., Christian, H. E., Friedmann, E., Taubert, K. A., ... Lange, R. A. (2013). Pet ownership and cardiovascular risk: A scientific statement from the American Heart Association. *Circulation, 127*(23), 2353–2363.

Martin, R. A., Graham, F. P., Taylor, W. J., & Levack, W. M. M. (2018). Mechanisms of change for children participating in therapeutic horse riding: A grounded theory. *Physical & Occupational Therapy in Pediatrics, 38*(5), 510–526.

McCardle, P., McCune, S., Griffin, J. A., Esposito, L., & Freund, L. (2010). *Animals in our lives: Human-Animal Interaction in Family, Community, & Therapeutic Settings*. Baltimore: Brookes.

McCardle, P., McCune, S., Griffin, J. A., Maholmes, V. (2010). *How animals affect us*. Washington, DC: American Psychological Association.

McColgan, G., & Schofield, I. (2007). The importance of companion animal relationships in the lives of older people. *Nursing Older People, 19*(1), 21–23.

McCune, S., Kruger, K. A., Griffin, J. A., Esposito, L., Freund, L. S., Hurley, K. J., & Bures, R. (2014). Evolution of research into the mutual benefits of human–animal interaction. *Animal Frontiers, 4*(3), 49–58.

McNicholas, J., & Collis, G. M. (2000). Dogs as catalysts for social interactions: Robustness of the effect. *British Journal of Psychology, 91*(1), 61–70.

McNicholas, J., Gilbey, A., Rennie, A., Ahmedzai, S., Dono, J. A., & Ormerod, E. (2005). Pet ownership and human health: A brief review of evidence and issues. *BMJ, 331*(7527), 1252–1254.

Melson, G. F. (2003). Child development and the human-companion animal bond. *American Behavioral Psychologist, 47*, 31–39.

Melson, G. F., & Fine, A. H. (2015). Animals in the lives of children. In *Handbook on animal-assisted therapy* (pp. 179–194). San Diego: Academic Press.

Mueller, M. K., Gee, N. R., & Bures, R. M. (2018). Human-animal interaction as a social determinant of health: Descriptive findings from the health and retirement study. *BMC Public Health, 18*(1), 305.

Nagengast, S., Baun, M., Megel, M., & Liebowitz, J. (1997). The effects of the presence of a companion animal of physiological arousal and behavioral distress in children. *Journal of Pediatric Nursing, 12*, 323–330.

O'Haire, M. O., McKenzie, S. J., McCune, S., & Slaughter, V. (2013). Effects of animal-assisted activities with Guinea Pigs in the Primary School Classroom. *Anthrozoos, 26*(3), 445–458.

Odendaal, J. S., & Meintjes, R. A. (2003). Neurophysiological correlates of affiliative behavior between humans and dogs. *Veterinary Journal, 165*(3), 296–301.

Ohtani, N., Kitagawa, K., Mikami, K., Kitawaki, K., Akiyama, J., Fuchikami, M., ... Ohta, M. (2017). horseback riding improves the ability to cause the appropriate action (go reaction) and the appropriate self-control (no-go reaction) in children. *Frontiers in Public Health, 5*, 8.

Parslow, R. A., Jorm, A. F., Christensen, H., Rodgers, B., & Jacomb, P. (2005). Pet ownership and health in older adults: Findings from a survey of 2,551 community-based Australians aged 60–64. *Gerontology, 51*(1), 40–47.

Pendry, P., Carr, A. M., Smith, A. N., & Roeter, S. M. (2014). Improving adolescent social competence and behavior: A randomized trial of an 11-week equine facilitated learning prevention program. *Journal of Primary Prevention, 35*(4), 281–293.

Pendry, P., Smith, A. N., & Roeter, S. M. (2014). Randomized trial examines effects of equine facilitated learning on adolescents' basal cortisol levels. *Human-Animal Interaction Bulletin, 2*(1), 80–95.

Redefer, L. A., & Goodman, J. F. (1989). Brief report: Pet-facilitated therapy with autistic children. *Journal of Autism Developmental Disorders, 19*(3), 461–467.

Reeves, M. J., Rafferty, A. P., Miller, C. E., & Lyon-Callo, S. K. (2011). The impact of dog walking on leisure-time physical activity: Results from a population-based survey of Michigan adults. *Journal of Physical Activity and Health, 8*(3), 436–444.

Rock, M., Mykhalovskiy, E., & Schlich, T. (2007). People, other animals and health knowledges: Towards a research agenda. *Social Science and Medicine, 64*(9), 1970–1976.

Sable, P. (1995). Pets, attachment, and well-being across the life cycle. *Social Work, 40*(3), 334–341.

Serpell, J., McCune, S., Gee, N., & Griffin, J. A. (2017). Current challenges to research on animal-assisted interventions. *Applied Developmental Science, 21*(3), 223–233. https://doi.org/10.1080/10888691.2016.1262775.

Stallones, L., Marx, M. B., Garrity, T. F., & Johnson, T. P. (1990). Pet ownership and attachment in relation to the health of US adults, 21 to 64 years of age. *Anthrozoös, 4*(2), 100–112.

Timperio, A., Salmon, J., Chu, B., & Andrianopoulos, N. (2008). Is dog ownership or dog walking associated with weight status in children and their parents? *Health Promotion Journal of Australia, 19*, 60–63.

Tourangeau, K., Nord, C., Lê, T., Wallner-Allen, K., Vaden-Kiernan, N., Blaker, L., & Najarian, M. (2018). *Early childhood longitudinal study, Kindergarten Class of 2010–11 (ECLS-K:2011) User's Manual for the ECLS-K:2011 Kindergarten–Fourth Grade Data File and Electronic Codebook, Public Version (NCES 2018-032)*. U.S. Department of Education. Washington, DC: National Center for Education Statistics.

Utz, R. L. (2014). Walking the dog: The effect of pet ownership on human health and health behaviors. *Social Indicators Research, 116*(2), 327–339.

Viau, R., Arsenault-Lapierre, G., Fecteau, S., Champage, N., Walker, C., & Lupien, S. (2010). Effect of service dogs on salivary cortisol secretion in autistic children. *Psychoneuroendocrinology, 35*(8), 1187–1193.

Wilson, C. (1987). Physiological responses of college students to a pet. *Journal of Nervous and Mental Diseases, 175*, 606–612.

Wood, L., Giles-Corti, B., & Bulsara, M. (2005). The pet connection: Pets as a conduit for social capital? *Social Science and Medicine, 61*, 1159–1173.

Wood, L., Martin, K., Christian, H., Nathan, A., Lauritsen, C., Houghton, S., … McCune, S. (2015). The pet factor-companion animals as a conduit for getting to know people, friendship formation and social support. *PloS ONE, 10*(4), e0122085.

Yamasaki, J. (2018). The communicative role of companion pets in patient-centered critical care. *Patient Education and Counseling, 101*(5), 830–835.

Zasloff, R. L. (1996). Measuring attachment to companion animals: A dog is not a cat is not a bird. *Applied Animal Behaviour Science, 47*(1–2), 43–48.

**Regina M. Bures, Ph.D.** is a Senior Program Director in the Population Dynamics Branch at the *Eunice Kennedy Shriver* National Institute of Child Health and Human Development (NICHD) at the National Institutes of Health. At NICHD, Dr. Bures manages a diverse scientific portfolio in demography and population health. She has been an active contributor to the NICHD-Waltham partnership. Dr. Bures received her Ph.D. in Sociology, with a specialization in Demography, from

Brown University and completed a postdoctoral fellowship at the University of Chicago. Dr. Bures has received numerous grants and awards, including research funding from the National Science Foundation and the National Institute of Aging. Her research interests include human-animal interaction, child and family health across the life course, data science, and research methods. She currently lives outside Washington, DC, with her husband, cats, dogs, and sheep.

**Layla Esposito, Ph.D., M.A.** is a program director in the Child Development and Behavior (CDB) Branch at the Eunice Kennedy Shriver National Institute of Child Health and Human Development (NICHD), National Institutes of Health (NIH) where she directs a program that includes research on social and emotional development in children and adolescents, child and family processes, human-animal interaction, and childhood obesity. Dr. Esposito completed her Ph.D. in social psychology and master's degree in clinical psychology at Virginia Commonwealth University. Prior to her position at NICHD, Dr. Esposito was a science policy fellow with the Society for Research in Child Development and the American Association for the Advancement of Sciences. Her prior research and clinical work focused on peer victimization, aggression, psychosocial functioning and adjustment in children, and child psychopathology.

**James A. Griffin, Ph.D.** is the Chief of the Child Development and Behavior Branch (CDBB) at the Eunice Kennedy Shriver National Institute of Child Health and Human Development (NICHD), National Institutes of Health (NIH), as well as the Director of the Early Learning and School Readiness Program. Prior to his position at NICHD, Dr. Griffin was a Senior Research Analyst in the Institute of Education Sciences (IES) at the U.S. Department of Education. He also served as the Assistant Director for the Social, Behavioral, and Education (SBE) Sciences in the White House Office of Science and Technology Policy (OSTP) and as a Research Analyst at the Administration on Children, Youth and Families (ACYF).

# Human-Animal Interaction and Child Health and Development

Megan K. Mueller

**Abstract** As pet ownership rates grow, the role of human-animal interaction (HAI) in promoting health and well-being of both human and animals is becoming an important area of public health research. In particular, it is important to explore the relationship between HAI and youth health and development. This chapter will explore how HAI fits into a framework of developmental science, and explore the theoretical underpinnings of youth-animal relationships. In addition, this chapter will review current research on HAI and youth social-emotional development, physical health, and cognition, and will also outline potential risks and challenges to child-pet interactions. Finally, we discuss research progress and future challenges within this area of child health and development.

**Keywords** Animal assisted therapy · Pet therapy · Stress reduction · Pets · Companion animals · Life course · Family life cycle · Child development · Caregiving · Stress · Aging · Health · Well-being · Bereavement · Human-animal interaction · Human-animal bond · Lifespan

Pets have become an increasingly important feature of family life, with upwards of two thirds of households in the United States reporting having at least one pet (American Pet Products Association, 2018). As discussed in chapter "Integrating Pets into the Family Life Cycle," companion animals are often viewed as members of the family (Cain, 1983; McConnell, Paige Lloyd, & Humphrey, 2019) and constitute an important relational component of family life (Mueller, Fine, & O'Haire, 2019). Given the status of pets in family life, it is important to explore how human-animal interaction (HAI) can contribute to child health and development. This chapter will discuss the role of pets as part of the developmental system for youth, the importance of understanding the complexities in these relationships, how HAI may be related to

---

M. K. Mueller (✉)
Cummings School of Veterinary Medicine, Tisch College of Civic Life, Tufts University, North Grafton, MA, USA
e-mail: megan.mueller@tufts.edu

social-emotional, cognitive, and physical outcomes, and potential risks that can be associated with companion animals.

## Pets in the Developmental System

The prevalence of pets, as well as the importance that humans place on these relationships, suggest that relationships with animals can be a particularly important component of the developmental system. Contemporary theoretical frameworks for understanding youth development are often framed using a relational, systems perspective (Overton, 2013) which suggests that child health and development should be viewed as the product of a multi-directional, integrated, dynamic relationship between the individual and the environmental context (Lerner, 2012). This type of theoretical framework is a useful tool for exploring the developmental processes involved in youth-animal relationships because it allows for the dynamic and often changing nature of relationships with pets. It also underscores the mutually-influential nature of child-animal relationships, highlighting the need to understand how interacting with pets may influence the health and well-being of the animals as well as the people involved in the interactions (Mueller, 2014a).

Conceptualizing human-animal interaction (HAI) as a component of the dynamic developmental system allows for research models that can assess the complexity of these relationships. Child-pet relationships are not static, and they may change over time as young people move through different developmental stages. Patterns of pet ownership in families vary based on age of children and socioeconomic and demographic characteristics (Westgarth et al., 2010), and children of different ages experience pet ownership in different ways (Hirschenhauser, Meichel, Schmalzer, & Beetz, 2017). Pet relationships contribute to developmental processes very early on; in infants as young as 10 months, there are differences between those with and without exposure to pets on visual inspection of animal faces (Hurley & Oakes, 2018). For a young child who is experiencing significant cognitive and language development, they may integrate the pet into these developmental tasks by talking about the animal (language practice), learning what their needs are (cognition), and experiencing the tactile nature of interacting with an animal (integration, self-regulation). In contrast, an adolescent who is working on fulfilling developmental goals of self-efficacy, social skills, and autonomy may have a more emotionally-connected relationship with a pet, using the relationship as a strategy for facilitating social relationships, practicing social skills, and exercising independence through caring for the animal. For example, pets can be a "social lubricant," fostering social connections between people as a common interest. Adolescence can also be a period of social transitions as peer group dynamics shift, and during this time, adolescents may rely on pets for nonjudgmental support in additional to physical comfort.

One of the most important aspects of child-pet interactions is understanding the quality and nature of these relationships. Not all relationships between children and pets are the same; there is significant diversity in biological, psychological, and social characteristics of both youth and animals, as well as past experiences that contribute to the shared relationship and potential outcomes. In particular, children's attachment to animals is an important component of understanding relationship quality in HAI. Children turn to their pets for emotional support during times of distress, which contributes to cognitive and emotional attachment (Covert, Whiren, Keith, & Nelson, 1985; Melson, Schwartz, & Beck, 1997). Attachment to pets is also dynamic, and there can be developmental differences in nature and strength of attachment as children age (Muldoon, Williams, Lawrence, & Currie, 2019). Although the research has been mixed, some recent work has found gender differences in attachment to pets, with girls reporting higher attachment than boys (Hawkins & Williams, 2017; Muldoon et al., 2019). These attachment relationships are an important component in shaping how children interact with pets. Youth who are attached to their pets may be more likely to engage with them on a regular basis, and therefore have the potential to further strengthen their bond.

Beyond attachment, which focuses primarily on the emotional component of youth-pet interactions, relationship quality can also include other types of relational engagement, including companionship, disclosure, relationship satisfaction (Cassels, White, Gee, & Hughes, 2017), and commitment to the relationship (Mueller, 2014b; Staats, Miller, Carnot, Rada & Turnes, 1996). Frequency and type of interactions are also important to measure, as there may be "dosage effects" of interacting with animals. For example, if there is a pet in the home that the child does not interact with, there is likely to be a differential impact compared to a pet with high levels of engagement. Furthermore, there are interactions with animals outside the home, and some animals participate in dual roles as both pet and part of an organized activity (e.g., 4-H, horseback riding). These different types of relationships may be associated with different types of developmental outcomes. For example, children who primarily interact with their pets in the home may have a more emotionally-oriented relationship, while those who participate in goal-directed activities with their animals may have interactions that foster specific skill-building.

Another aspect of this relationship is how a child conceptualizes an individual animal or groups of animals. For example, higher levels of belief about animal minds (e.g., that animals are sentient and have thoughts and feelings) were shown to be related to higher attachment to pets and animals, positive attitudes about animals, compassion, and caring behaviors towards animals, and lower levels of acceptance towards animal cruelty and neglect (Hawkins & Williams, 2016). Furthermore, this study showed that children with pets had higher levels of belief of animal minds, suggesting that pet relationships may contribute to children's views on animals more broadly. There is also significant evidence that youth have different relationships with different species of animals, even within the same household (with children often reporting higher levels of attachment to dogs), further supporting the notion that each individual relationship should be considered as part of the complex developmental system (Cassels et al., 2017; Hawkins & Williams, 2016, 2017; Mueller, 2014c; Muldoon et al., 2019).

Attachment, relationship quality, and how youth view animals are particularly important components of understanding how HAI can contribute (both positively and negatively) to child health and development. These measures have often been more useful predictors of developmental outcomes as compared to pet ownership alone (e.g., Jacobson & Chang, 2018; Mueller, 2014b). Similar to other types of interpersonal relationships, the mere presence of a pet may not matter as much as the nature of that interaction within the developmental system, including how the individual relationship between a child and a pet may interact with other relationships in the family (e.g., siblings, parents), as well as broader factors such as socioeconomic status, community setting, and cultural attitudes about animals. All these factors must be considered when conducting and interpreting research exploring the health and developmental outcomes associated with HAI.

## Social-Emotional Development

Given the diverse relationships children and adolescents have with animals, pets are uniquely positioned within the developmental system to potentially contribute to multiple domains of functioning, including social-emotional development. As previously noted, many children have social relationships with animals, which, under the right circumstances, can provide the opportunity to develop positive social and emotional skills. Empathy and prosocial behaviors are often cited as outcomes linked with pets, driven by the hypothesis that caring for an animal may support social skills by facilitating social relationships, building a foundation for the development of social competence, and fostering perspective-taking that can lead to empathic behaviors. For example, caring for a pet may allow children to understand the individual needs of a pet, and how those needs differ from their own, setting the stage for developing the reciprocal behaviors that are a key aspect of moral development. Some existing research has supported HAI as an aspect of social developmental processes, demonstrating associations between attachment and positive attitudes towards pets and empathy, social connections, social competence, and prosocial behavior (Jacobson & Chang, 2018; Mueller, 2014c; Poreskey & Hendrix, 1989). However, as noted in a recent review by Purewal et al. (2017), other research has found null or negative associations between pet ownership and social development outcomes (Mathers, Canterford, Olds, Waters, & Wake, 2010; Vidović, Štetić, & Bratko, 1999). These mixed results underscore that the way in which children interact with pets matters, as well as the need for understanding the varied nature of these relationships. For young people who do not engage regularly or in social or caretaking capacities with their pets, they may not have the opportunity to practice the behaviors involved in adaptive social skills. Understanding the nature and quality of child-pet relationships is critical in identifying when and how pets can promote social development.

Although relatively understudied in youth, there is some initial evidence that adolescents who own pets are less lonely than non-pet owners, and that attachment to animals may be related to a more robust social support network (Black, 2012). Attachment to a pet may also serve as an emotional buffer during times of stress and has been associated with the utilization of adaptive social coping skills (Mueller & Callina, 2014). Pet relationships may provide a way for youth to process their emotions during times of stress as a "safe" outlet for emotional disclosure. When peer conflict leads to loneliness, an adaptive relationship with an animal may provide some of the social support that a youth needs to cope with this conflict. Animal relationships may also serve as a social bridge for facilitating peer or family relationships within the developmental system. For example, pets can be an entry point into conversation with a peer around a shared interest (e.g., discussing one's pets) that can create a pathway to a relationship. Pet caretaking tasks, such as dog walking, can also be a regular way in which children can interact positively with their parents or siblings. However, the nature of these specific relational processes has not been fully explored in the research.

A related component of healthy social development for youth is adaptive self-regulation skills (Diener & Kim, 2004; Gestsdóttir & Lerner, 2007). The ability to successfully regulate emotions and cope with distress, conflict, and arousal are key components of social-emotional development, and there is increasing evidence that these skills can be fostered through HAI (Flynn, Mueller, Luft, Geldhof, Klee, Tedeschi, & Morris, 2020; Kršková, Talarovic̆ová, & Olexová, 2010). In addition to emotional support, physical contact with animals may have a physiological effect of reducing arousal and anxiety (Ein, Li, & Vickers, 2018; Kerns, Stuart-Parrigon, Coifman, van Dulmen, & Koehn, 2018; Polheber & Matchock, 2014; Vormbrock & Grossberg, 1988), which promotes the conditions necessary for adaptive emotional regulation. When a child is able to regulate their arousal, they are better able to control their emotions, even in challenging circumstances.

Similarly, some of the same processes associated with adaptive self-regulation may also promote social anxiety reduction more broadly. For adolescents in particular, social anxiety is a specific concern as the most common anxiety disorder (Bogels et al., 2010; Heimberg, Stein, Hiripi, & Kessler, 2000), with onset of social anxiety disorder most often occurring during the adolescent years (Otto, Pollack, Maki, Gould, Worthington, Smoller, & Rosenbaum, 2001). An adolescent-animal relationship can become part of the that person's representation of social resources, which may reduce the perception of social risk and lead to decreased anxiety. For example, the knowledge that they can rely on the pet as a safe, consistent, and nonjudgmental source of emotional support can provide a buffer for feeling anxious about social relationships or conflicts. Some recent evidence has shown that during a social stressor, the presence of a pet dog can in fact buffer perceived social stress (Kertes et al., 2017) and support positive affect (Kerns et al., 2018), providing support for this hypothesis.

It should be noted that many of the positive associations between HAI and positive social behaviors are related to attachment and/or attitudes towards pets, and the presence of a pet in the home without a measure of relational quality appears to be a less robust predictor of positive outcomes. These findings underscore the need for exploring the quality and features of youth-pet relationships in the context of positive developmental outcomes, particularly when social in nature. Furthermore, much of the research that has been done in this area is not causal, and future research should explore directionality in these relationships. For example, it may be that youth who have more robust social networks and enhanced social skills are better able to connect with pets, creating a positive feedback loop of social behaviors. It is very challenging to establish causal relationships between pets and social outcomes, because of the non-random nature of who owns pets. For the vast majority of families, they elect to have a pet, and reasons they decide to get a pet may confound any potential effects. For example, a family who has stable, strong social relationships with little maladaptive conflict may be more likely to feel they have the capacity to have a companion animal. Therefore, it is difficult to determine if better social-emotional outcomes are due to the presence of a pet, or other characteristics within the family setting. In the absence of randomized controlled trials (which are challenging due to the logistical and ethical issues with randomly assigning pets to families) or other large scale, population-representative longitudinal research studies, the existing research base has not yet definitely established causal relationships between pets and social-emotional outcomes for young people.

## Cognition

From a very young age, exposure to pets is related to infant cognition, and specifically to face recognition (Hurley & Oakes, 2018). Beyond infancy, a significant body of research has suggested that the presence of an animal (and dogs in particular) can improve cognitive skills, which in turn are predictive of academic success (Gee & Fine, 2019). One hypothesized developmental process underpinning these findings is that animals may help children focus their attention, which improves performance in cognitive tasks. For example, it has been demonstrated that children who perform motor skills tasks in the presence of a dog compared to a human, complete the tasks faster without sacrificing accuracy (Gee, Belcher, Grabski, DeJesus, & Rile, 2012; Gee, Church, & Altobelli, 2010), and they require fewer instructional prompts to complete the tasks (Gee, Crist, & Carr, 2010). Similar results have been found for children when asked to perform cognitive tasks such as categorization or memory tasks (Gee & Fine, 2019), with performance improvements in both tasks in the presence of a real dog compared to a stuffed/toy dog. More recent research from two large scale randomized controlled trials has shown a positive relationship between interacting with a dog and improved executive functioning in 8-10 children (Brelsford, Meints, & Gee, Under Review) and college students (Pendry, Carr, & Gee, Under Review). Executive functioning is a cluster of important cognitive processes such as working memory, planning, and inhibition that are all positive correlated with success in life. The effects seen in these studies are still present after a longitudinal delay and may ultimately lead us to the conclusion that interacting with a dog is associated with success in life. More research is needed, but the results are certainly provocative and suggest that interactions with animals should be explored within the context of cognitive development.

## Physical Health

In addition to socioemotional and cognitive development, one hypothesized health effect of HAI is physical well-being. Particularly regarding physical activity and healthy body weight, it has been hypothesized that exercising or being active with a pet (e.g., dog walking) may be a particularly motivating and engaging way for children to stay active. However, the association between pet ownership and physical activity for children has been mixed. The majority of positive links between pet ownership and physical health are related to dog ownership (given that dogs are more easily incorporated into physical activities compared to smaller pets such as guinea pigs, fish, or even cats), with some research finding that children who live with a dog are more likely to be physically active and less likely to be overweight (Timperio, Salmon, Chu, & Andrianopoulos, 2008). However, other research has found no differences in childhood obesity based on dog ownership (Westgarth et al., 2012), or that positive health effects associated with pet ownership are attenuated when other demographic factors are controlled for (Miles, Parast, Babey, Griffin, & Saunders, 2017).

Interpreting the relationship between pets and physical health is likely complicated by significant selection factors, and as previously noted, randomized controlled trials are rare due to the practical and ethical concerns with randomly assigning families to pet ownership. In particular, it has been documented that there are significant differences between families that do and do not own pets on a number of variables that may be related to physical health, including income level, age, and having parents who are in good health and employed (Adhikari et al., 2019; Marsa-Sambola et al., 2016; Miles et al., 2017; Westgarth et al., 2010). Therefore, it is unclear if children who are in families who are already more active and healthier are more likely to get a pet (and a pet who can engage in physical activity), if the pet causes some change in these behaviors, or a combination of both. In addition, the role of relationship quality is important to explore; Linder and colleagues (2017) found that overweight youth had higher levels of attachment to their pets and lower levels of perceived human social support than youth who were not overweight, suggesting that a supportive relationship with a pet might be particularly important for overweight children and adolescents.

Similarly, there is some limited evidence that dog walking and other similar intervention programs can help foster physical activity for young people (Westgarth et al., 2013). Other programs have found that such programs for youth are met with high levels of enthusiasm and acceptability with the intervention but limited significant impact on physical health outcomes (Morrison et al., 2013). Additional research in this area of health outcomes is needed to fully elucidate the impact of HAI on physical activity, nutrition, and healthy body rate, including what types of pets and interactions with pets might be related to physical health.

While less explored, it has also been suggested that there may be a relationship between pets and prevalence of allergies in youth. Hölscher, Frye, Wichmann, and Heinrich (2002) found a protective relationship between contact with dogs during the first year of life and lifetime prevalence of asthma, hay fever, itchy rash, and pollen sensitization (although these results were not seen with other types of pets), and similar relationships have been replicated for asthma and eczema (Pohlabeln, Jacobs, & Böhmann, 2007), and allergic family history (Eller et al., 2008). In contrast, other studies have found no association between pet exposure and allergic sensitization or asthma (Carlsen et al., 2012; Miles et al., 2017; Torrent et al., 2007; Wegienka et al., 2010). It is important to point out that if a child displays allergic symptoms in reaction to a pet, the parents may opt to remove the pet from the home, systematically changing their status from pet owner to non-pet owner. This simple action commonly taken by parents can make a sample of pet owners appear to look as if it contains fewer allergic symptoms/diagnoses relative to a sample of non-pet owners, making it difficult to establish causality

## Potential Risks and Challenges

While pets often make a positive contribution to the developmental system, HAI is not without risks to child health. Animals are living creatures with their own sets of behaviors and needs, which can sometimes be in conflict with child behaviors. One potential risk is bite-related injuries, particularly with dogs (Meints, Racca, & Hickey, 2010). Children often have difficulty correctly interpreting dogs' facial expressions and general signs of stress and discomfort, which is a risk factor for injury (Meints et al., 2010). In particular, young children often incorrectly identify fearful dogs, and therefore are more likely to approach them (Aldridge & Rose, 2019). Further complicating this problem, adults also have difficulty identifying fear and anxiety in dogs during dog-child interaction, which is a barrier to preventing situations that can lead to a bite injury (Demirbas et al., 2016). There have been a number of programs designed to address bite prevention, such as "The Blue Dog" Bite Prevention Program (Meints & de Keuster, 2009). Several reviews of such prevention programs have found them to be moderately effective, but compliance is challenging (Schwebel, Li, McClure, & Severson, 2016; Shen, Rouse, Godbole, Wells, Boppana, & Schwebel, 2017) and children need consistent reminding about safe behaviors around dogs (Meints, Brelsford, & De Keuster, 2018). Engaging parents in supporting safe interactions between children and pets (particularly for younger children) is a critical component in preventing injuries and animal stress.

Beyond direct physical risks, it is important to understand some of the other types of challenges that can be associated with pet interactions. Caring for a pet requires some investment of time and monetary resources. Estimates have suggested a financial cost of $10,000 or more during the lifetime of a dog (Ingram, 2019), although these costs can vary widely based on a number of factors, including species (e.g., horse versus fish) and geographic location. While the caretaking aspect of pet ownership can be considered an opportunity for skill-building for children, it may also cause stress within the family system, particularly if combined with other emotional, financial, and time pressures. Pets can also get sick, which presents significant financial costs in terms of veterinary care as well as emotional challenges, and can contribute to caregiver burden and stress (Spitznagel, Mueller, Frachak, Hoffman, & Carlson, 2019). Therefore, understanding the "goodness-of-fit" between a particular pet and a family system is a critical component of fostering adaptive human-animal interaction. There may be characteristics of both the individual animals and their preferences, constellation of the family (number of people and number of animals), and type and age of children, that can all contribute to compatibility (Hart et al., 2018).

In addition to risks to humans, the well-being of companion animals is an equally important consideration. Children have varying levels of experience and views on understanding what their own pets might need (Muldoon, Williams, & Lawrence, 2016). Therefore, appropriate adult supervision is needed to ensure that individual animals are having their basic physical and behavioral needs met within a family. Age-appropriate monitoring of child-animal interactions, routines, and animal behavior are all important components of maintaining positive interactions, and this structure may be particularly important for families with children with developmental challenges (Hall, Wright, & Mills, 2017). Maintaining positive interactions is critical, as the animals often bear the majority of the consequences of negative events.

## Research Issues and Challenges

Significant progress has been made over the last decade with regard to research quality within the field of human-animal interaction more broadly, including the increased use of rigorous designs such as randomized controlled trials, larger sample sizes, and validated measures (McCune et al., 2019). One area of particular growth is the development of measurement approaches that are specifically designed to measure human-animal relationships (see Gee & Schulenburg, 2017 for a review of measures). These include self-report measures that can be included in survey or intervention research (e.g., Cassels et al., 2017; Bures, Mueller, & Gee, 2019), as well as observational measures that provide more objective quantification of HAI (Guérin et al., 2018). There has also been increased use of physiological measures such as cortisol, oxytocin, and heart rate which provide a more robust understanding of the complex biopsychosocial processes involved in HAI (Beetz, Uvnas-Moberg, Julius, & Kotrschal, 2012; Kertes et al., 2017; Pan, Granger, Guérin, Shoffner, & Gabriels, 2018). The expanding availability of measures that have been validated for use specifically in human-animal interaction has significantly increased the quality of research data.

However, there are still significant limitations in our current understanding of HAI and youth development. Much of the existing research on child-animal interaction is still cross-sectional, and the lack of longitudinal research limits our current understanding about if and how human-animal relationships may impact long-term health and behavior for young people. As previously noted, there are practical and ethical issues associated with randomly assigning pet ownership, and therefore existing HAI research is limited by selection effects regarding who chooses to own a pet (and what kind of pet), how different sociodemographic factors predict whether families get or keep pets, and how these factors may mediate or moderate any outcomes associated with pet ownership (Miles et al., 2017). These limitations translate to a relative lack of understanding about the details of for whom, and under what circumstances, pet ownership is beneficial. More robust datasets are needed to identify and explore the individual, contextual, and environmental factors that may influence the relationship between pets and socio-emotional and physical well-being.

In particular, the interaction between cultural identity, social environment, and companion animals has been significantly understudied in HAI research. The majority of existing HAI research has been conducted with relatively affluent populations with limited racial/ethnic and cultural diversity, limiting generalizability about findings related to attitudes towards animals. Despite cultural differences in attitudes towards pets, little research exists exploring how cultural and racial/ethnic identity may influence the relationship between pets and developmental outcomes. In order to understand for which families having a pet may be beneficial, there is a need for research that includes comprehensive measures of cultural and ethnic identity. In addition, pets are an important feature of the social environment within family and community settings (Wood, Giles-Corti, & Bulsara, 2005; Wood et al., 2015). However, few existing studies include robust indicators of within-family features (such as parental monitoring and family conflict) as well as broader contextual features such as neighborhood characteristics that are important potential mediators of the relationship between pets and health outcomes.

To overcome these challenges in existing HAI research and more fully understand the role of pet ownership as a contextual predictor of social-emotional and physical health for youth, there is a significant need for integrating HAI measures into population-based, nationally-representative studies that are specifically designed to characterize social and emotional development in adolescence, as well as other types of study designs that can obtain longitudinal, developmentally-relevant data. Pet relationships are just one component of the complex developmental system, and interactions between youth and animals do not exist in a vacuum. It is likely that HAI may be a moderating or mediating factor in many other processes within the developmental system, and therefore research should treat these relationships with according complexity. Furthermore, mental and physical health practitioners should consider asking about pets as an important component of understanding the full functioning of the family system.

## Conclusions

Human-animal interaction has the potential to significantly impact a wide range of domains of child health and development, and therefore is an important area of scholarly inquiry that has implications for public health. However, children's relationships with companion animals can be complex, and are embedded in the larger developmental system, which includes integration with the family, community, and broader ecological systems. Therefore, there is a need for rigorous approaches to research that measure the nuances of HAI and can connect these relationships to broader systems of health. By better understanding the role of HAI in child health and development, families, practitioners, educators, and other youth-serving professionals will be able to maximize the potential contribution of these relationships for youth. Furthermore, by understanding the nuances of child-animal relationships, we can promote well-being and quality of life for the animals in our lives.

# References

Adhikari, A., Wei, Y., Jacob, N., Hansen, A. R., Snook, K., Burleson, C. E., & Zhang, J. (2019). Association between pet ownership and the risk of dying from colorectal cancer: An 18-year follow-up of a national cohort. *Journal of Public Health*, 1–8.

Aldridge, G. L., & Rose, S. E. (2019). Young children's interpretation of dogs' emotions and their intentions to approach happy, angry, and frightened dogs. *Anthrozoös, 32*(3), 361–374.

American Pet Products Manufacturers Association (APPA). (2018). *2017–2018 APPA National Pet Owners Survey*. Retrieved from http://www.americanpetproducts.org/press_industrytrends.asp.

Beetz, A., Uvnäs-Moberg, K., Julius, H., & Kotrschal, K. (2012). Psychosocial and psychophysiological effects of human-animal interactions: The possible role of oxytocin. *Frontiers in Psychology, 3,* 234. https://doi.org/10.3389/fpsyg.2012.00234.

Black, K. (2012). The relationship between companion animals and loneliness among rural adolescents. *Journal of Pediatric Nursing, 27*(2), 103–112.

Bogels, S. M., Alden, L., Beidel, D. C., Clark, L. A., Pine, D. S., Stein, M. B., & Voncken, M. (2010). Social anxiety disorder: Questions and answers for the DSM-V. *Depression and Anxiety, 27*(2), 168–189.

Brelsford, V., Meints, K., & Gee, N. R. (Under Review). Effects of animal-assisted interventions on executive functioning in school children. *International Journal of Environmental Research and Public Health*.

Bures, R. M., Mueller, M. K., & Gee, N. R. (2019). Measuring human-animal attachment in a large U.S. survey: Two brief measures for children and their primary caregivers. *Frontiers in Public Health (Human-Animal Interaction [HAI] Research: A Decade of Progress), 7*, 107. https://doi.org/10.3389/fpubh.2019.00107.

Cain, A. O. (1983). A study of pets in the family system. In A. H. Katcher & A. M. Beck (Eds.), *New perspectives on our lives with companion animals* (pp. 72–81). Philadelphia: University of Pennsylvania Press.

Carlsen, K. C. L., Roll, S., Carlsen, K. H., Mowinckel, P., Wijga, A. H., Brunekreef, B., ... Krämer, U. (2012). Does pet ownership in infancy lead to asthma or allergy at school age? Pooled analysis of individual participant data from 11 European birth cohorts. *PloS One, 7*(8), e43214.

Cassels, M. T., White, N., Gee, N., & Hughes, C. (2017). One of the family? Measuring young adolescents' relationships with pets and siblings. *Journal of Applied Developmental Psychology, 49,* 12–20.

Covert, A. M., Whiren, A. P., Keith, J., & Nelson, C. (1985). Pets, early adolescents, and families. *Marriage & Family Review, 8*(3–4), 95–108.

Demirbas, Y. S., Ozturk, H., Emre, B., Kockaya, M., Ozvardar, T., & Scott, A. (2016). Adults' ability to interpret canine body language during a dog–child interaction. *Anthrozoös, 29*(4), 581–596.

Diener, M. L., & Kim, D. Y. (2004). Maternal and child predictors of preschool children's social competence. *Journal of Applied Developmental Psychology, 25*(1), 3–24.

Ein, N., Li, L., & Vickers, K. (2018). The effect of pet therapy on the physiological and subjective stress response: A meta-analysis. *Stress and Health, 34*(4), 477–489.

Eller, E., Roll, S., Chen, C. M., Herbarth, O., Wichmann, H. E., Von Berg, A., ... Brunekreef, B. (2008). Meta-analysis of determinants for pet ownership in 12 European birth cohorts on asthma and allergies: A GA2LEN initiative. *Allergy, 63*(11), 1491–1498.

Flynn, E., Mueller, M. K., Luft, D., Geldhof, G. J., Klee, S., Tedeschi, P., & Morris, K. N. (2020). Human-animal-environment interactions and self-regulation in youth with psychosocial challenges: Initial assessment of the Green Chimneys model. *Human-Animal Interaction Bulletin, 8*(2), 53–65.

Gee, N. R., Belcher, J., Grabski, J., DeJesus, M., & Riley, W. (2012). The presence of a therapy dog results in improved object recognition performance in preschool children. *Anthrozoös, 25,* 289–300.

Gee, N. R., Church, M. R., & Altobelli, C. L. (2010). Preschoolers make fewer errors on an object categorization task in the presence of a dog. *Anthrozoös, 23,* 223–230.

Gee, N. R., Crist, E. N., & Carr, D. N. (2010). Preschool children require fewer instructional prompts to perform a memory task in the presence of a dog. *Anthrozoös, 23,* 178–184.

Gee, N. R., & Fine, A. H. (2019). Animals in educational settings: Research and practice. In A. H. Fine (Ed.), *Handbook on animal-assisted therapy: Theoretical foundations and guidelines for applying animal assisted interventions* (5th ed., pp. 271–284). Amsterdam: Elsevier.

Gee, N. R., & Schulenburg, A. N. (2017). Recommendations for measuring the impact of animals in education settings. In N. R. Gee, A. H. Fine, & P. McCardle (Eds.), *How Animals Help Students Learn: Research and Practice for Educators and Mental-Health Professionals* (pp. 157–181). New York, NY: Routledge Publishers, Taylor & Francis Group.

Gestsdóttir, S., & Lerner, R. M. (2007). Intentional self-regulation and positive youth development in early adolescence: Findings from the 4-H study of youth development. *Developmental Psychology, 43*(2), 508–521. https://doi.org/10.1037/-12-1649.43.2.508.

Guérin, N. A., Gabriels, R. L., Germone, M. M., Schuck, S. E., Traynor, A., Thomas, K. M., ... O'Haire, M. E. (2018). Reliability and validity assessment of the Observation of Human-Animal Interaction for Research (OHAIRE) behavior coding tool. *Frontiers in Veterinary Science, 5.* http://doi.org/10.3389/fvets.2018.00268.

Hall, S. S., Wright, H. F., & Mills, D. S. (2017). Parent perceptions of the quality of life of pet dogs living with neuro-typically developing and neuro-atypically developing children: An exploratory study. *PLoS ONE, 12*(9), e0185300.

Hart, L. A., Hart, B. L., Thigpen, A. P., Willits, N. H., Lyons, L. A., & Hundenski, S. (2018). Compatibility of Cats with Children in the Family. *Frontiers in Veterinary Science, 5:* 278. http://doi.org/10.3389/fvets.2018.00278.

Hawkins, R. D., & Williams, J. M. (2016). Children's beliefs about animal minds (Child-BAM): Associations with positive and negative child–animal interactions. *Anthrozoös, 29*(3), 503–519.

Hawkins, R., & Williams, J. (2017). Childhood attachment to pets: Associations between pet attachment, attitudes to animals, compassion, and humane behaviour. *International Journal of Environmental Research and Public Health, 14*(5), 490.

Heimberg, R. G., Stein, M. B., Hiripi, E., & Kessler, R. C. (2000). Trends in the prevalence of social phobia in the United States: A synthetic cohort analysis of changes over four decades. *European Psychiatry, 15,* 29–37.

Hirschenhauser, K., Meichel, Y., Schmalzer, S., & Beetz, A. M. (2017). Children love their pets: Do relationships between children and pets co-vary with taxonomic order, gender, and age? *Anthrozoös, 30*(3), 441–456.

Hölscher, B., Frye, C., Wichmann, H. E., & Heinrich, J. (2002). Exposure to pets and allergies in children. *Pediatric Allergy and Immunology, 13*(5), 334–341.

Hurley, K., & Oakes, L. M. (2018). Infants' daily experience with pets and their scanning of animal faces. *Frontiers in Veterinary Science, 5,* 152.

Ingram, C. (2019, November 22). Researchers have finally put a price tag on the life of a dog. *The Washington Post.* Retrieved from https://www.washingtonpost.com/business/2019/11/22/researchers-have-finally-put-price-tag-life-dog/.

Jacobson, K. C., & Chang, L. (2018). Associations between pet ownership and attitudes toward pets with youth socioemotional outcomes. *Frontiers in Psychology, 9*, 2304.

Kerns, K. A., Stuart-Parrigon, K. L., Coifman, K. G., van Dulmen, M. H., & Koehn, A. (2018). Pet dogs: Does their presence influence preadolescents' emotional responses to a social stressor? *Social Development, 27*(1), 34–44.

Kertes, D. A., Liu, J., Hall, N. J., Hadad, N. A., Wynne, C. D., & Bhatt, S. S. (2017). Effect of pet dogs on children's perceived stress and cortisol stress response. *Social Development, 26*(2), 382–401.

Kršková, L., Talarovičová, A., & Olexová, L. (2010). Guinea pigs—The "small great" therapist for autistic children, or: Do guinea pigs have positive effects on autistic child social behavior? *Society & Animals, 18*(2), 139–151.

Lerner, R. M. (2012). Developmental science, developmental systems, and contemporary theories of human development. In W. Damon & R. M. Lerner (Eds.), *Handbook of child psychology* (pp. 1–17). New York: Wiley.

Linder, D. E., Sacheck, J. M., Noubary, F., Nelson, M. E., & Freeman, L. M. (2017). Dog attachment and perceived social support in overweight/obese and healthy weight children. *Preventive Medicine Reports, 6*, 352–354.

Marsa-Sambola, F., Williams, J., Muldoon, J., Lawrence, A., Connor, M., Roberts, C., … Currie, C. (2016). Sociodemographics of pet ownership among adolescents in Great Britain: Findings from the HBSC Study in England, Scotland, and Wales. *Anthrozoös, 29*(4), 559–580.

Mathers, M., Canterford, L., Olds, T., Waters, E., & Wake, M. (2010). Pet ownership and adolescent health: Cross-sectional population study. *Journal of Paediatrics and Child Health, 46*(12), 729–735.

McConnell, A. R., Paige Lloyd, E., & Humphrey, B. T. (2019). We are family: Viewing pets as family members improves wellbeing. *Anthrozoös, 32*(4), 459–470.

McCune, S., Kruger, K. A., Griffin, J. A., Esposito, L., Bures, R. M., Hurley, K. J., & Gee, N. R. (2019). Strengthening the foundation of human-animal interaction research: Recent developments in a rapidly growing field. In A. H. Fine (Ed.), *Handbook on animal-assisted therapy: Theoretical foundations and guidelines for applying animal assisted interventions* (5th ed., pp. 487–497). Amsterdam: Elsevier.

Meints, K., Brelsford, V., & De Keuster, T. (2018). Teaching children and parents to understand dog signalling. *Frontiers in Veterinary Science, 5*, 257.

Meints, K., & de Keuster, T. (2009). Brief Report: Don't kiss a sleeping dog: The first assessment of "The Blue Dog" Bite Prevention Program. *Journal of Pediatric Psychology, 34*(10), 1084–1090.

Meints, K., Racca, A., & Hickey, N. (2010). How to prevent dog bite injuries? Children misinterpret dogs' facial expression. *Injury Prevention, 16*, A68.

Melson, G. F., Schwartz, R. I., & Beck, A. M. (1997). Importance of companion animals in children's lives: Implications for veterinary practice. *Journal of the American Veterinary Medical Association, 211*(12), 1512–1518.

Miles, J. N., Parast, L., Babey, S. H., Griffin, B. A., & Saunders, J. M. (2017). A propensity-score-weighted population-based study of the health benefits of dogs and cats for children. *Anthrozoös, 30*(3), 429–440.

Morrison, R., Reilly, J. J., Penpraze, V., Westgarth, C., Ward, D. S., Mutrie, N., … Yam, P. S. (2013). Children, parents and pets exercising together (CPET): Exploratory randomised controlled trial. *BMC Public Health, 13*(1), 1096.

Mueller, M. K. (2014a). Human-animal interaction (HAI) as a context for positive youth development: A relational developmental systems approach to constructing HAI theory and research. *Human Development, 57*(1), 5–25.

Mueller, M. K. (2014b). Is human-animal interaction (HAI) linked to positive youth development? Initial answers. *Applied Developmental Science, 18*(1), 5–16.

Mueller, M. K. (2014c). The relationship between types of human-animal interaction and emotions and cognitions about animals: An exploratory study. *Anthrozoös, 27*(2), 295–308.

Mueller, M. K., & Callina, K. S. (2014). Human–animal interaction as a context for thriving and coping in military-connected youth: The role of pets during deployment. *Applied Developmental Science, 18*(4), 214–223.

Mueller, M. K., Fine, A. H., & O'Haire, M. E. (2019). Understanding the role of human-animal interaction in the family context. In A. H. Fine (Ed.), *Handbook on animal-assisted therapy: Theoretical foundations and guidelines for applying animal assisted interventions* (5th ed., pp. 351–362). Amsterdam: Elsevier.

Muldoon, J. C., Williams, J. M., & Lawrence, A. (2016). Exploring children's perspectives on the welfare needs of pet animals. *Anthrozoös, 29*(3), 357–375.

Muldoon, J. C., Williams, J. M., Lawrence, A., & Currie, C. (2019). The nature and psychological impact of child/adolescent attachment to dogs compared with other companion animals. *Society & Animals, 27*(1), 55–74.

Overton, W. F. (2013). A new paradigm for developmental science: Relationism and relational-developmental systems. *Applied Developmental Science, 17*(2), 94–107.

Otto, M. W., Pollack, M. H., Maki, K. M., Gould, R. A., Worthington, J. J., Smoller, J. W., & Rosenbaum, J. F. (2001). Childhood history of anxiety disorders among adults with social phobias: Rates, correlates, and comparisons with patients with panic disorder. *Depression and Anxiety, 14*(4), 209–213.

Pan, Z., Granger, D. A., Guérin, N. A., Shoffner, A., & Gabriels, R. L. (2018). Replication pilot trial of therapeutic horseback riding and cortisol collection with children on the autism spectrum. *Frontiers in Veterinary Science, 5.* http://doi.org/10.3389/fvets.2018.00312.

Pendry, P., Carr, A. M., & Gee, N. R. (Under Review). Randomized controlled trial examining effects of varying levels of Human-Animal Interaction and risk-status on students' executive function in a University based Animal Visitation Program (AVP).

Pohlabeln, H., Jacobs, S., & Bohmann, J. (2007). Exposure to pets and the risk of allergic symptoms during the first 2 years of life. *Journal of Investigational Allergology and Clinical Immunology, 17*(5), 302–308.

Polheber, J. P., & Matchock, R. L. (2014). The presence of a dog attenuates cortisol and heart rate in the Trier Social Stress Test compared to human friends. *Journal of Behavioral Medicine, 37*(5), 860–867.

Poresky, R. H., & Hendrix, C. (1989). Companion animal bonding, children's home environments, and young children's social development. In *Proceedings of the 21st National Biennial Meeting of the Society for Research in Child Development.* Kansas City, MO.

Purewal, R., Christley, R., Kordas, K., Joinson, C., Meints, K., Gee, N., & Westgarth, C. (2017). Companion animals and child/adolescent development: A systematic review of the evidence. *International Journal of Environmental Research and Public Health, 14*(3), 234.

Schwebel, D. C., Li, P., McClure, L. A., & Severson, J. (2016). Evaluating a website to teach children safety with dogs: A randomized controlled trial. *International Journal of Environmental Research and Public Health, 13*(12), 1198.

Shen, J., Rouse, J., Godbole, M., Wells, H. L., Boppana, S., & Schwebel, D. C. (2017). Systematic review: Interventions to educate children about dog safety and prevent pediatric dog-bite injuries: A meta-analytic review. *Journal of Pediatric Psychology, 42*(7), 779–791.

Spitznagel, M. B., Mueller, M. K., Fraychak, T., Hoffman, A. H., & Carlson, M. D. (2019). Validation of a brief assessment of caregiver burden in clients with an ill companion animal. *Journal of Veterinary Internal Medicine, 33*(3), 1251–1259. https://doi.org/10.1111/jvim.15508.

Staats, S., Miller, D., Carnot, M. J., Rada, K., & Turnes, J. (1996). The Miller-Rada commitment to pets scale. *Anthrozoös, 9*(2–3), 88–94.

Timperio, A., Salmon, J., Chu, B., & Andrianopoulos, N. (2008). Is dog ownership or dog walking associated with weight status in children and their parents? *Health Promotion Journal of Australia, 19*(1), 60–63.

Torrent, M., Sunyer, J., Garcia, R., Harris, J., Iturriaga, M. V., Puig, C., … Cullinan, P. (2007). Early-life allergen exposure and atopy, asthma, and wheeze up to 6 years of age. *American Journal of Respiratory and Critical Care Medicine, 176*(5), 446–453.

Vidović, V. V., Štetić, V. V., & Bratko, D. (1999). Pet ownership, type of pet and socio-emotional development of school children. *Anthrozoös, 12*(4), 211–217.

Vormbrock, J. K., & Grossberg, J. M. (1988). Cardiovascular effects of human-pet dog interactions. *Journal of Behavioral Medicine, 11*(5), 509–517.

Westgarth, C., Boddy, L. M., Stratton, G., German, A. J., Gaskell, R. M., Coyne, K. P., ... Dawson, S. (2013). A cross-sectional study of frequency and factors associated with dog walking in 9–10 year old children in Liverpool, UK. *BMC Public Health, 13*(1), 822.

Westgarth, C., Heron, J., Ness, A. R., Bundred, P., Gaskell, R. M., Coyne, K. P., ... Dawson, S. (2010). Family pet ownership during childhood: Findings from a UK birth cohort and implications for public health research. *International Journal of Environmental Research and Public Health, 7*(10), 3704–3729.

Westgarth, C., Heron, J., Ness, A. R., Bundred, P., Gaskell, R. M., Coyne, K., ... Dawson, S. (2012). Is childhood obesity influenced by dog ownership? No cross-sectional or longitudinal evidence. *Obesity Facts, 5*(6), 833–844.

Wood, L., Giles-Corti, B., & Bulsara, M. (2005). The pet connection: Pets as a conduit for social capital? *Social Science and Medicine, 61,* 1159–1173. https://doi.org/10.1016/j.socscimed.2005.01.017.

Wood, L., Martin, K., Christian, H., Nathan, A., Lauritsen, C., Houghton, S., ... McCune, S. (2015). The pet factor-companion animals as a conduit for getting to know people, friendship formation and social support. *PloS ONE, 10*(4), e0122085.

**Megan K. Mueller, Dr.** is the Elizabeth Arnold Stevens Junior Professor and Assistant Professor of human-animal interaction at the Cummings School of Veterinary Medicine at Tufts University, and Co-Director of the Tufts Institute for Human-Animal Interaction. She is also a senior fellow at the Jonathan M. Tisch College of Civic Life at Tufts University and teaches in the M.S. in Animals and Public Policy program at the Center for Animals and Public Policy. Dr. Mueller is a developmental psychologist, and her research program focuses on assessing the effects of pet ownership and animal-assisted interventions on adolescent development and family functioning. In particular, her work focuses on how HAI can support youth with social anxiety and promote thriving in adolescence. Her research has been funded by the National Institutes of Health (NIH), and private foundations, and her work has been published in numerous scientific journals and media outlets. She is also a board member of Tufts Paws for People, a Pet Partners Community Partner therapy animal group.

# Successful Aging and Human-Animal Interaction

Nancy R. Gee

**Abstract** Adults over the age of 65 now represent a substantially larger proportion of the US population than ever before and the percentage of older adults is on the rise. Advancing age is commonly associated with a number of mental and physical health risks including reduced social networks, and increased risk of mortality and morbidity. As the population of older adults increases so will the demand on the health care system which makes it increasingly important to find ways to support healthy or successful aging. This chapter discusses the potential of companion animals to address, at least in part, this growing concern. This chapter will summarize some of the key research findings suggesting that companion animals may play a role in promoting healthy active aging and will briefly discuss the physical and mental health benefits associated with pet ownership or with the simple act of interacting with a companion animal.

**Keywords** Animal assisted therapy · Pet therapy · Stress reduction · Pets · Companion animals · Life course · Family life cycle · Child development · Caregiving · Stress · Aging · Health · Well-being · Bereavement · Human-animal interaction · Human-animal bond · Lifespan

## Pet Ownership and Older Adults

The proportion of adults over the age of 65 has been on the increase since 1950 when it was a mere 8% of the US population. That number has increased to 16% today and is projected to increase to 26% by 2050 (https://www.prb.org/agingpopulationclocks/). Commonly accompanying advancing age are a number of health risks including decreased cognitive and physical functioning, along with reduced social networks, and increased risk of mortality and morbidity (Friedmann et al., 2020). As the population of older adults increases so will the demand on the health care system

---

N. R. Gee (✉)
Center for Human-Animal Interaction, School of Medicine, Virginia Commonwealth University, Richmond, VA, USA
e-mail: Nancy.Gee@VCUHealth.org

© The Author(s), under exclusive license to Springer Nature Switzerland AG 2021
R. Bures et al., *Well-Being Over the Life Course*,
SpringerBriefs in Well-Being and Quality of Life Research,
https://doi.org/10.1007/978-3-030-64085-9_6

which makes it increasingly important to find ways to support healthy or successful aging. The goal of successful aging is to live the highest quality life for as long as possible. There is an accumulation of evidence suggesting that companion animals may play a role in promoting healthy active aging, and this chapter will summarize the latest available science on this subject. We will discuss the physical and mental health benefits associated with pet ownership or with the simple act of interacting with an animal.

Pet ownership is very common among older adults, with 89% of adults over the age of 50 reporting that they have kept a pet at some point in their lives (Friedmann et al., 2019). Not surprisingly, the two most commonly cited reasons for owning a pet are enjoyment and companionship. Despite the fact that dog ownership has been associated with a lower risk of death over the long term and thus positively associated with survival (Kramer, Mehmood, & Suen, 2019), the data are showing that pet ownership decreases with advancing age (Friedmann et al., 2019). This pattern of decreasing pet ownership appears to follow similar general patterns of age-related declines in cognitive function, physical function, and psychological status, suggesting that maintaining ones' pet may become increasingly challenging with advancing age.

## *Physical Health and Exercise*

Evidence of the positive effects of pet ownership on physical health occurs principally in two areas: cardiac health and stress responses, and increased physical activity, particularly in the form of dog walking. Owning a pet has been found to be a predictor of survival for older adults with a history of cardiac events or conditions. Among 460 individuals who had experienced a myocardial infarction, only pet ownership was found to be a significant factor associated with survival (Friedmann, Thomas, & Son, 2011). In a sample of hypertensive older adults, those owning pets had improved survival rates and a lower risk of fatal cardiovascular events (Chowdhury et al., 2017).

When 191 older adults suffering typical age-related health problems (diabetes, hypertension and/or hyperlipidemia) were fitted with Holter monitors over a 24-h period, the presence of their pets modulated the cardiac autonomic imbalances in their electrocardiogram results (Aiba et al., 2012). Similarly, the presence of their pets was associated with lower blood pressure in 32 hypertensive older adult patients (Friedmann, Thomas, Son, Chapa, & McCune, 2013). Although their comments were not restricted to older adults, the American Heart Association issued an important scientific statement in 2013 indicating that pet ownership, particularly dog ownership, may reduce risk for cardiovascular disease (Levine et al., 2013). Further, they suggest that there may be a causal relationship such that owning a dog may be causally connected to reducing ones' risk of cardiovascular disease.

More studies have examined the effect of pet ownership on physical activity. The benefits of regular walking for seniors are many-fold: a reduction in heart disease, high blood pressure, stroke and cholesterol; improvement in muscle strength and balance; calorie reduction; mood improvement through endorphin release; and social engagement (Nelson et al., 2007; Pedersen & Saltin, 2006; Roberts & Barnard, 2005).

Although older adults are more likely to adhere to a walking regime than other forms of exercise (Masuki et al., 2014), it is nevertheless still true that overall physical activity decreases with age, and that older adults are the most sedentary segment of the population (Dall et al., 2017). Multiple studies have shown that older adult dog owners engage in significantly more walking than non-pet owners (Dall et al., 2017; Dembicki & Anderson, 1996; Feng et al., 2014; Garcia et al., 2015; Harris, Owen, Victor, Adams, & Cook, 2009; Shibata et al., 2012; Thorpe, Kreisle et al., 2006; Thorpe, Simonsick et al., 2006), helping this group achieve the recommended 150 min per week of physical activity (US Dept of HHS, 2018; WHO, 2011). Whether these older adults walk their dogs out of a feeling of obligation to provide them with exercise, because they simply enjoy spending time with them, because dog-walking creates an excuse to get out of the house, or for some other reason isn't always evident, but whatever the reason, the humans benefit by increasing their activity level.

To the last point on the benefits-of-walking list, a 2013 random survey of nearly 900 older adults found that those who frequently walked their dogs felt a higher sense of community (Toohey, McCormack, Doyle-Baker, Adams, & Rock, 2013). The perceptions of older adults regarding the benefits of their companion animals, communicated in focus groups (Knight & Edwards, 2008), paralleled the results of these studies, as they indicated that they accrued both health and social benefits from dog walking.

Not all research addressing pet ownership and health has found the relationship to be positive. In a study of 242 patients admitted to a hospital for acute cardiac symptoms, pet owners, especially cat owners, were more likely to suffer mortality or hospital re-admission (Parker et al., 2010). Another survey of 2,551 older adults comparing pet owners and non-owners found that those who cared for a pet had lower physical health (Parslow, Jorm, Christensen, Rodgers, & Jacomb, 2005). Some studies found no difference on various measures of physical health, positive or negative, between older adults who owned pets and those who did not (Crowley-Robinson & Blackshaw, 1998; Winefield, Black, & Chur-Hansen, 2008). Results also vary across species: in two studies where cat ownership was negatively associated with health outcomes, dog ownership was positively linked. We simply do not have enough data to make strong claims about different species of pets, because most of the research related to human-animal interaction is conducted on dogs.

The factors affecting the impact of pet ownership on the physical health of older adults are complex. To gain a more complete picture we must find ways to determine, for instance, whether persons who are already healthy and/or economically secure are more likely to own and walk pets than those who are less fortunate on either count. Looking at the same question from another angle, if we can resolve some of the challenges to pet ownership for older adults, will health benefits begin to accrue?

## *Mental Health*

Despite numerous studies in the literature, the relationship between pet ownership and mental health for older adults remains unclear. An early study found that pet ownership/attachment was associated with less depression in 1,232 bereaved adults over the age of 65 (Garrity, Stallones, Marx, & Johnson, 1989). However, since then a number of studies have found no relationship between pet ownership and depression in older adults (Antonacopoulos & Pychyl, 2010; Branson, Boss, Cron, & Kang, 2016; Miller & Lago, 1990), while other research has associated pet ownership with higher rates of depression (Mueller, Gee, & Bures, 2018; Parslow et al., 2005). Unfortunately, these latter studies are based on cross-sectional analyses of large databases and are thus not subject to causal interpretation. Similar to our efforts to understand the potential physical health benefits of pet ownership, we need to tease out the whether pet ownership triggers depression or simply doesn't relieve it, or whether depressed individuals are more likely to acquire a pet as a potential method of "self-treatment", than are others. This will require more sophisticated design and analysis on the part of researchers, but a better understanding of this relationship is most certainly warranted.

## *Loneliness*

A key concern for our aging population among both physical and mental health practitioners is loneliness and social isolation, and a number of studies have found positive relationships between pet ownership and attenuated loneliness. As noted above, older adults in a focus group indicated that dog-walking increased their social interactions (Knight & Edwards, 2008). Pet attachment has been associated with lower loneliness in older adults (Krause-Parello & Gulick, 2013) and with mediating the relationship between loneliness and general health (Krause-Parello, 2008). A survey of 814 adults over 60 living alone found that pets were effective in moderating loneliness (Stanley, Conwell, Bowen, & Van Orden, 2014), and a probability sample of 298 rural adults in the same age range identified an association between pet ownership and self-esteem/locus of control, though only for men (Hecht, McMillin, & Silverman, 2001).

Similar to the case with depression, it is possible that acquiring a pet may be perceived as a means of coping with loneliness (Krause-Parello, 2012). One study found that pet owners were more likely to have fewer friends than non-pet owners, suggesting that a lack of a robust social network may lead to the acquisition of a pet for companionship (Stewart, Thrush, Paulus, & Hafner, 1985).

The authors of a study of 5,210 English older adults found that pet owners were significantly more likely to report loneliness than non-owners, and suggest that gender differences could be responsible, since women are both more likely to be pet owners and to report loneliness (Pikhartova, Bowling, & Victor, 2014). They further speculate that, for women, pet ownership may be "both a response to loneliness and a potential pathway out of loneliness" (p. 9).

Other studies have found no differences in loneliness or social support attributable to pet ownership (Antonacopoulos & Pychyl, 2010; Bennett, Trigg, Godber, & Brown, 2015; Eshbaugh et al., 2011; Winefield et al., 2008). The relationships between and among pets, loneliness and aging are clearly complex. Prior ownership of a pet, attachment to current and prior pets, the species of pet, the gender and economic circumstances of the owner—these and other factors must be explored more thoroughly before any statements regarding the circumstances under which pet ownership can attenuate loneliness can be stated with confidence, but the results of these studies are encouraging and suggest that future research on the topic of loneliness should consider pet ownership as an important variable of study.

## Interacting with Companion Animals

It is interesting to note that regular contact with pets has been linked to better verbal memory regardless of age (Friedmann et al., 2020), and that many older adults (37%) who are not pet owners report having regular contact with pets. This regular contact may come in the form of interacting with the pets owned by family members, or it may be the result of planned and structured animal-assisted activities or interventions. Collectively these are known as Animal Assisted Interactions ("AAI"). Those that are more casual are generally classed as Animal Assisted Activities ("AAA"), while those that are intended as goal-oriented therapy sessions and are delivered by trained professionals (with training typically required of any animals (usually dogs) that are involved) are known as Animal Assisted Therapy ("AAT"). Although most research is conducted using AAT, the benefits may appear through AAA as well.

### *Physical Health and Exercise*

It is typically easier to conduct robust analyses of the effects of companion animals on humans via animal assisted interventions than pet ownership, given the challenges of establishing control conditions by randomly assigning pets to owners. People tend to want to select their own pet (e.g., dog, cat) rather than have one assigned to them (e.g., horse, bird). Experimentally controlled conditions also make it more straightforward to manipulate the details of the presence of the animal (e.g., when, where and how often) and then to measure psychological or physiological responses to the presence of the animal.

In a well-designed study from 2007, a group of older adults with advanced heart failure who received visits from a volunteer/dog team benefited more on a number of measures than parallel groups who were visited by only a volunteer or did not receive visits (Cole, Gawlinski, Steers, & Kotlerman, 2007). Both during and after the visit, the volunteer/dog group had significantly greater decreases in systolic blood pressure assessments, in epinephrine and norepinephrine, and in anxiety.

In another randomized control trial involving dogs and older adults published that same year, participants' blood pressure was found to be significantly lower when they were asked to speak in the presence of a dog than when they were asked to speak when the dog was absent (Friedmann, Thomas, Cook, Tsai, & Picot, 2007). There was no difference in blood pressure when the participants were simply sitting, not speaking. The sample size was small and the results should be interpreted with some caution, but the study was well planned and executed, and the authors' point that an accumulation of small reductions in blood pressure throughout a day can yield health benefits certainly contributes to our understanding of how the presence of a pet may impact the health of older adults.

The Pet Assisted Living (PAL) study compared physical activity between two groups of mildly cognitively impaired older adults following two forms of interactions with visiting dogs (Friedmann et al., 2015). In the PAL condition, the participants performed specific skills with the dogs, such as petting or brushing, and in the comparison condition, participants were encouraged to look at photos and reminisce about events earlier in their lives. The PAL group improved significantly more in measures of physical activity than the reminiscing group. Again, however, the sample size was relatively small so we should be cautious in our conclusions, but the results are certainly encouraging and indicative of the need for further exploration of the important role that dogs may play when interacting with older adult in an assisted living setting.

A number of less rigorous studies have reported that AAI reduced the potential for falls in older adults (Araujo, Silva, Costa, Pereira, & Safons, 2011), as well as reducing blood pressure, hospitalization, and other stress indicators (Krause-Parello & Kolassa, 2016; Sloane, Zimmerman, Gruber-Baldini, & Barba, 2002; Stasi et al., 2004). In addition to these results, other studies, while plagued by design or size limitations, have reported increased walking speed or ability, improved balance and stability, and increased nutritional intake in response to AAI (Edwards & Beck, 2002, 2013; Harris, Rinehart, & Ge, 1993; Luptak & Nuzzo, 2004; Nordgren & Engström, 2012; Rondeau et al., 2010; Walsh, Mertin, Verlander, & Pollard, 1995; Wehofer, Goodson, & Shurtleff, 2013). And moving away from dogs and cats, viewing an aquarium has been found to result in decreased heart rate, muscle tension and skin temperature (DeSchriver & Riddick, 1990).

## Mental Health

Overall, most studies on AAI in this area indicate a positive impact of AAI on mental health, specifically depression. Korean researchers were able to randomly and temporarily assign pets (crickets) to one group of participants in their study (Ko, Youn, Kim, & Kim, 2016). Both this group and the control group were subject to psychometric and laboratory tests at the beginning of the study period and again at the conclusion, both groups were provided guidance on healthy lifestyle choices, and both groups had ongoing contact with research assistants. At the end of 8 weeks, the cricket-carers had significantly improved depression and cognition scores when compared with the control group, although there was no difference in other measures (anxiety, stress, fatigue, insomnia, inflammatory markets). The use of insects may be culturally bound and thus not generalizable, but the study is encouraging in its exploration of the potential benefits of caring for pets generally, and for specifically caring for pets that do not require walking or emptying litter boxes.

Other studies report beneficial effects of AAI on depression. In one where groups of cognitively intact older adults were randomly assigned to either a canary, a plant, or a blank control over a period of 3 months, the canary group showed greater improvement in depression and quality of life scores than either of the other two conditions (Colombo, Buono, Smania, Raviola, & DeLeo, 2006). Another randomized control trial involved 55 mild to moderately cognitively impaired older adults in an assisted living environment (Travers, Perkins, Rand, Bartlett, H., Morton, 2013). The participants were assigned to either dog-assisted or human-only therapy over a period of 11 weeks, after which the dog-assisted therapy group had significantly improved depression/quality of life scores when compared with the human-only group. Most other similar studies showed reductions in depression associated with AAI (Friedmann et al., 2015; Kumasaka, Masu, Kataoka, & Numao, 2012; LeRoux & Kemp, 2009; Mossello et al., 2011; Stasi et al., 2004), although some showed no changes (Barker, Pandurangi, & Best, 2003; Francis, Turner, & Johnson, 1985; Lutwack-Bloom, Wijewickrama, & Smith, 2005; Zisselman, Rovner, Shmuely, & Ferrie, 1996).

Much of the research on depression and AAI also addresses anxiety; given the established connection between depression and anxiety (Gorman, 1996), measures of anxiety are frequently included in the psychological assessment tools used for or with depression. There is less consistency in the results of the studies evaluating the impact of AAI on anxiety than on depression, however. Although an AAI session reduced anxiety in patients with advanced heart failure in the Cole et al. study referenced above (Cole et al., 2007), and also in 10 Alzheimer's patients (Mossello et al., 2011), the same effect was not present in a study of 16 long term care facility residents (LeRoux & Kemp, 2009). In other studies AAI has been seen to reduce behavior problems that may be related to anxiety or agitation (Dabelko-Schoeny et al., 2014; Edwards, Beck, & Lim, 2014; McCabe, Baun, Speich, & Agrawal, 2002; Sellers, 2005). Barker et al. compared the effects of 15 min spent with magazines versus 15 min spent with therapy dogs on anxiety, fear and depression prior to electroconvulsive therapy for 35 adults with serious mental health problems. The therapy dog condition produced significant reductions in fear, though not in anxiety or depression (Barker et al., 2003).

Because neither the treatments nor the methodologies employed by either the depression or anxiety studies are consistent, and most of the studies have been small in scale and of a short term, it is difficult to draw any meaningful conclusions in terms of what works, what doesn't, and why. As with so many other aspects of AAI, only more well-designed and targeted research following up on these studies will provide that information. However, this accumulation of evidence does give us leave to presume that there may in fact be a link between pet interaction and reductions in both depression and anxiety. We must leave it to future research to establish a causal link, and to help us to clearly understand the when, where, and why pet interactions may ameliorate depression and possible anxiety.

## *Loneliness*

Presumably because AAI can be seen as a potential prescription to reduce loneliness and social isolation, there has been more research in this area than in any other aspect of AAI as it affects older adults. Most of these studies have reported positive effects of AAI on loneliness, although some found no effect at all.

In one of the larger studies, 45 residents of a long-term care facility were assigned at random to either a once-per-week AAT group, a 3 times-per-week AAT group, or a no AAT group (Banks & Banks, 2002). Both AAT groups had greater reductions in loneliness after 6 weeks than the no AAT control group. The individuals who opted to participate in the study had life-long histories and emotional connections with pets, raising the important question: is it a prior relationship with pets that makes AAT helpful in reducing loneliness? A similar result was found in a study by Vrbanac et al. (2013), which assessed the impact of AAT on loneliness in 21 nursing home residents over six months. The results were again positive, and again, most of the participants had previously owned a pet. The impact of prior pet ownership on outcomes will be an important topic for future research if we are to determine the ways in which companion animals can be optimally employed to address the loneliness among older adults.

Other studies, smaller and observational, have found increases in social interactions associated with AAI, suggesting a parallel reduction in loneliness. The populations studied have included older psychiatric patients, dementia sufferers, retirement home, long-term care and nursing home residents, and community dwellers (Fick, 1993; Haughie, 1992; Katsinas, 2000; Koda & Yanai, 2011; Kongable, Buckwalter, & Stolley, 1989; Kramer, Friedmann, & Bernstein, 2009; Krause-Parello & Kolassa, 2016; Marx et al., 2010; Sellers, 2005). The increased socializations have been among residents/patients and also between residents/patients and staff. As noted, some studies reported no significant differences between AAI group and non-AAI groups, but none described a negative effect.

As was the case above, we will leave it to future researchers to help us sort out the details of when, where and why pets may be most effective at combatting loneliness for older adults, but the findings to-date are very encouraging. It seems that for those people who desire, or enjoy, or have a history of pet ownership, interacting with animals does alleviate their loneliness. It is worth pausing to consider precisely what that means. Loneliness and social isolation are reaching epidemic proportions and the negative effects on health and wellbeing are well described. If companion animals may alleviate loneliness or social isolation, even in a sub-group of older adults, that is worth noting.

## Conclusion and Next Steps

In sum, although the research to date into the impact of pet ownership and AAI on physical health, mental health and loneliness is promising, more consistency in methodology, intervention strategies, measurement techniques, and implementations, along with larger study populations, will be needed to support meaningful conclusions that can be interpreted on a large scale. Even so, the evidence to date is both promising and exciting. We have good reason to suspect that pet interaction especially, and some aspects of pet ownership, are likely to have positive physical and mental health outcomes for older adults. The future is bright for researchers interested in this topic, as they are likely to make major discoveries about the circumstances under which pets may improve the lives of older adults.

With that said, it is of paramount importance to consider the animal side of this topic. When therapy animals are involved animal assisted interactions, the handler is present to see to the needs, both emotional and physical, of the animal involved. The handler typically owns the animal, most commonly a dog, and is responsible for their immediate and long-term care, so risks to the animal are minimal and addressed immediately by the handler/owner. However, a number of concerns may arise when we address the issue of older adults owning pets. In most cases, older adults are capable and responsible pet owners, but if or when an older adult suffers a health problem, or when the pet may become ill and requires potentially expensive veterinary care, older adults may require support to responsibly maintain their pet in their home. In some cases, an older adult may forego their own medical treatment if they do not have access to pet care because they are concerned that an extended hospital stay will require them to give up their animal. In other cases, an older adult with declining cognition may not fully understand or be able to implement the daily duties required of responsible pet ownership. In one case, the human's health may suffer and in the other case, the pet's health may suffer. Both situations are unacceptable and rather than take the obvious and blunt step of removing the animal, we should consider finding ways to support older adults in both responsible self-care and responsible pet ownership without the older adult experiencing a looming fear of becoming separated from their beloved pet.

There are a number of next steps that we can take to support older adults continued ownership or interaction with companion animals. For example, if we improved companion animal access to public transportation that would make it much easier and more cost-effective for pet owners of all ages to take their pet to the veterinarian and other service locations, and it would also make it easier for therapy dog handlers to travel to the homes of older adults to provide in-home visits with their dogs. An all-too-common reason that older adults give up their pets is that they may need to move into an assisted-living environment, and in many cases, these housing situations do not allow for pets. We need to take the step of improving companion animal access to housing of all types, but especially assisted living or nursing home facilities. Finally, we need to find ways to get the community involved in supporting older adults in maintaining their pets. For example, there are unique programs in which college students, who are away from home and their pets, are matched with older adult pet owners. Together they work out a schedule in which the college student may do simple pet related tasks such as walking the dog or cleaning the litter tray to help support an older adult who may be dealing with a mobility issue. In this example, both the student and the older adult benefit from this pairing.

These ideas represent the beginning of how we might be able to support older adults in either owning or interacting with companion animals. AAI is inexpensive and the research is showing a number of psychological and physical health benefits for older adults. It is time to recognize the importance and potential life changing impact of AAI for older adults who enjoy pets. AAI may not be effective for all older adults, but for those who desire it, there is no reason not to make it a regular part of their lives.

## References

Aiba, N., Hotta, K., Yokoyama, M., Wang, G., Tabata, M., Kamiya, K., ... Masuda, T. (2012). Usefulness of pet ownership as a modulator of cardiac autonomic imbalance in patients with diabetes mellitus, hypertension, and/or hyperlipidemia. *American Journal of Cardiology, 109*, 1164–1170.

Antonacopoulos, N. M. D., & Pychyl, T. A. (2010). An examination of the potential role of pet ownership, human social support and pet attachment in the psychological health of individuals living alone. *Anthrozoös, 23*, 37–54.

Araujo, T. B., Silva, N. A., Costa, J. N., Pereira, M. M., & Safons, M. P. (2011). Effect of equine-assisted therapy on the postural balance of the elderly. *Brazilian Journal of Physical Therapy, 15*, 414–419.

Banks, M. R., & Banks, W. A. (2002). The effects of animal-assisted therapy on loneliness in an elderly population in long-term care facilities. *Journal of Gerontology, 57A*, M428–M432.

Barker, S. B., Pandurangi, A., & Best, A. M. (2003). Effects of animal-assisted therapy on patients' anxiety, fear, and depression before EDT. *The Journal of ECT, 19*, 38–44.

Bennett, P. C., Trigg, J. L., Godber, T., & Brown, C. (2015). An experience sampling approach to investigating associations between pet presence and indicators of psychological wellbeing and mood in older Australians. *Anthrozoös, 28*, 403–420.

Branson, S., Boss, L., Cron, S., & Kang, D.-H. (2016). Examining differences between homebound older adult pet owners and non-pet owners in depression, systemic inflammation, and executive function. *Anthrozoös, 29*, 323–334.

Chowdhury, E. K., Nelson, M. R., Jennings, G. L., Wing, L. M., Reid, C. M., & ANBP2 Management Committee. (2017). Pet ownership and survival in the elderly hypertensive population. *Journal of Hypertension, 35*, 769–775.

Cole, K. M., Gawlinski, A., Steers, N., & Kotlerman, J. (2007). Animal-assisted therapy in patients hospitalized with heart failure. *American Journal of Critical Care, 16*, 575–588.

Colombo, G., Buono, M. D., Smania, K., Raviola, R., & DeLeo, D. (2006). Pet therapy and institutionalized elderly: A study on 144 cognitive unimpaired subjects. *Archives of Gerontology and Geriatrics, 42*, 207–216.

Crowley-Robinson, P., & Blackshaw, J. K. (1998). Pet ownership and health status of elderly in the community. *Anthrozoös, 11*, 168–171.

Dabelko-Schoeny, H., Phillips, G., Darrough, E., DeAnna, S., Jarden, M., Johnson, D., & Lorch, G. (2014). Equine-assisted intervention for people with dementia. *Anthrozoös, 27*, 141–155.

Dall, P. M., Ellis, S. L. H., Ellis, B. M., Grant, P. M., Colyer, A., Gee, N. R., & Mills, D. S. (2017). The influence of dog ownership on objective measures of free-living physical activity and sedentary behaviour in community- dwelling older adults: A longitudinal case-controlled study. *BMC Public Health, 17,* 496. https://doi.org/10.1186/s12889-017-4422-5.

Dembicki, D., & Anderson, J. (1996). Pet ownership may be a factor in improved health of the elderly. *Journal of Nutrition for the Elderly, 15,* 15–31.

DeSchriver, M. M., & Riddick, C. C. (1990). Effects of watching aquariums on elders' stress. *Anthrozoös, 4,* 44–48.

Edwards, N. E., & Beck, A. M. (2002). Animal-assisted therapy and nutrition in Alzheimer's disease. *Western Journal of Nursing Research, 24,* 697–712.

Edwards, N. E., & Beck, A. M. (2013). The influence of aquariums on weight in individuals with dementia. *Alzheimer Disease and Associated Disorders, 27,* 379–383.

Edwards, N. E., Beck, A. M., & Lim, E. (2014). Influence of aquariums on resident behavior and staff satisfaction in dementia units. *Western Journal of Nursing Research, 36,* 1309–1322.

Eshbaugh, E. M., Somervill, J. W., Kotek, J. H., Perez, E., Nalan, K. R., & Wilson, C. E. (2011). Presence of a dog, pet attachment, and loneliness among elders. *North American Journal of Psychology, 13*(1), 1–4.

Feng, Z., Dibben, C., Witham, M. D., Donnan, P. T., Vadiveloo, T., Sniehotta, F., & McMurdo, M. E. (2014). Dog ownership and physical activity in later life: A cross-sectional observational study. *Preventive Medicine, 66,* 101–106.

Fick, K. M. (1993). The influence of an animal on social interactions of nursing home residents in a group setting. *American Journal of Occupational Therapy, 47,* 529–534.

Francis, G., Turner, J. T., & Johnson, S. B. (1985). Domestic animal visitation as therapy with adult home residents. *International Journal of Nursing Studies, 22,* 201–206.

Friedmann, E., Galik, E., Thomas, S. A., Hall, P. S., Chung, S. Y., & McCune, S. (2015). Evaluation of a pet-assisted living intervention for improving functional status in assisted living residents with mild to moderate cognitive impairment: A pilot study. *American Journal of Alzheimer's Disease & Other Dementias, 30,* 276–289.

Friedmann, E., Gee, N. R., Simonsick, E. M., Studenski, S., Barr, E., Resnick, B., … Hackney, A. (2019). Pet ownership patterns and successful aging outcomes in community dwelling older adults. *Frontiers in Veterinary Science, 7,* 293.

Friedmann, E., Thomas, S. A., Cook, L. K., Tsai, C., & Picot, S. J. (2007). A friendly dog as potential moderator of cardiovascular response to speech in older hypertensives. *Anthrozoös, 20,* 51–63.

Friedmann, E., Thomas, S. A., & Son, H. (2011). Pets, depression and long-term survival in community living patients following myocardial infarction. *Anthrozoös, 24,* 273–285.

Friedmann, E., Thomas, S. A., Son, H., Chapa, D., & McCune, S. (2013). Pet's presence and owner's blood pressures during the daily lives of pet owners with pre- to mild hypertension. *Anthrozoös, 26,* 535–550.

Garcia, D. O., Wertheim, B. C., Manson, J. E., Chlebowski, R. T., Volpe, S. L., Howard, B. V., & Thomson, C. A. (2015). Relationships between dog ownership and physical activity in postmenopausal women. *Preventive Medicine, 70,* 33–38.

Garrity, T. F., Stallones, L., Marx, M. B., & Johnson, T. P. (1989). Pet ownership and attachment as supportive factors in the health of the elderly. *Anthrozoös, 3,* 35–44.

Gorman, J. M. (1996). Comorbid depression and anxiety spectrum disorders. *Depression and Anxiety, 4,* 160–168.

Harris, M. D., Rinehart, J. M., & Gerstman, J. (1993). Animal-assisted therapy for the homebound elderly. *Holistic Nursing Practice, 8,* 27–37.

Harris, T. J., Owen, C. G., Victor, C. R., Adams, R., & Cook, D. G. (2009). What factors are associated with physical activity in older people, assessed objectively by accelerometry? *British Journal of Sports Medicine, 43,* 442–450. https://doi.org/10.1136/bjsm.2008.048033.

Haughie, E. (1992). An evaluation of companion pets with elderly psychiatric patients. *Behavioural Psychotherapy, 20,* 367–371.

Hecht, L., McMillin, D., & Silverman, P. (2001). Pets, networks, and wellbeing. *Anthrozoös, 14,* 95–108.

Katsinas, R. P. (2000). The use and implications of a canine companion in a therapeutic day program for nursing home residents with dementia. *Activities, Adaptation & Aging, 25,* 13–30.

Knight, S., & Edwards, V. (2008). In the company of wolves: The physical, social, and psychological benefits of dog ownership. *Journal of Aging and Health, 20,* 437–455.

Ko, H. J., Youn, C. H., Kim, S. H., & Kim, S. Y. (2016). Effect of pet insects on the psychological health of community-dwelling elderly people: A single-blinded, randomized, controlled trial. *Gerontology, 62,* 200–209.

Koda, N., & Yanai, J. (2011). Dog—Resident interactions in a Japanese retirement home. *Anthrozoös, 24,* 155–165.

Kongable, L. G., Buckwalter, K. C., & Stolley, J. M. (1989). The effects of pet therapy on the social behavior of institutionalized Alzheimer's clients. *Archives of Psychiatric Nursing, 3,* 191–198.

Kramer, C. K., Mehmood, S., & Suen, R. S. (2019, October). Dog ownership and survival: A systematic review and meta-analysis. *Circulation: Cardiovascular Quality and Outcomes.* https://doi.org/10.1161/circoutcomes.119.005554.

Kramer, S. C., Friedmann, E., & Bernstein, P. L. (2009). Comparison of the effect of human interaction, animal—Assisted therapy, and AIBO-assisted therapy on long-term care residents with dementia. *Anthrozoös, 22,* 43–57.

Krause-Parello, C. A. (2008). The mediating effect of pet attachment support between loneliness and general health in older females living in the community. *Journal of Community Health Nursing, 25,* 1–14.

Krause-Parello, C. A. (2012). Pet ownership and older women: The relationships among loneliness, pet attachment support, human social support, and depressed mood. *Geriatric Nursing, 33,* 194–203.

Krause-Parello, C. A., & Gulick, E. E. (2013). Situational factors related to loneliness and loss over time among older pet owners. *Western Journal of Nursing Research, 35,* 905–919.

Krause-Parello, C. A., & Kolassa, J. (2016). Pet therapy: Enhancing social and cardiovascular wellness in community dwelling older adults. *Journal of Community Health Nursing, 33,* 1–10.

Kumasaka, T., Masu, H., Kataoka, M., & Numao, A. (2012). Changes in patient mood through animal-assisted activities in a palliative care unit. *International Medical Journal, 19,* 373–377.

LeRoux, M., & Kemp, R. (2009). Effect of a companion dog on depression and anxiety levels of elderly residents in a long-term care facility. *Psychogeriatrics, 9,* 23–26.

Levine, G., Allen, K., Braun, L. T., Christian, H. E., Friedmann, E., Taubert, K. A., ... Lange, R. A. (2013). Pet ownership and cardiovascular risk: A scientific statement from the American Heart Association. *Circulation, 127,* 2353–2363.

Luptak, J. E., & Nuzzo, N. A. (2004). The effects of small dogs on vital signs in elderly women: A pilot study. *Cardiopulmonary Physical Therapy Journal, 15,* 9–12.

Lutwack-Bloom, P., Wijewickrama, R., & Smith, B. (2005). Effects of pets versus people visits with nursing home residents. *Journal of Gerontological Social Work, 44,* 137–159.

Marx, M. S., Cohen-Mansfield, J., Regier, N. G., Dakheel-Ali, M., Srihari, A., & Thein, K. (2010). The impact of different dog-related stimuli on engagement of persons with dementia. *American Journal of Alzheimer's Disease & Other Dementias, 25,* 37–45.

McCabe, B. W., Baun, M. M., Speich, D., & Agrawal, S. (2002). Resident dog in the Alzheimer's special care unit. *Western Journal of Nursing Research, 24,* 684–696.

Masuki, S., Mori, M., Tabara, Y., Sakurai, A., Hashimoto, S., Morikawa, M., ... Nose, H. (2014). The factors affecting adherence to a long-term interval walking training program in middle-aged and older people. *Journal of Applied Physiology, 118*(5), 595–603.

Miller, M., & Lago, D. (1990). The wellbeing of older women: The importance of pet and human relations. *Anthrozoös, 3,* 245–252.

Mossello, E., Ridolfi, A., Mello, A. M., Lorenzini, G., Mugnai, F., Piccini, C., ... Marchionni, N. (2011). Animal–assisted activity and emotional status of patients with Alzheimer's disease in day care. *International Psychogeriatrics, 23,* 899–905.

Mueller, M. K., Gee, N. R., & Bures, R. M. (2018). Human–animal interaction as a social determinant of health: Descriptive findings from the Health and Retirement Study. *BMC Public Health, 18,* 305. https://doi.org/10.1186/s12889-018-5188-0.

Nelson, M. E., Rejeski, W. J., Blair, S. N., Duncan, P. W., Judge, J. O., King, A. C., ... Castaneda-Sceppa, C. (2007). Physical activity and public health in older adults: recommendation from the American College of Sports Medicine and the American Heart Association. *Circulation, 116*(9), 1094.

Nordgren, L., & Engström, G. (2012). Effects of animal-assisted therapy on behavioral and/or psychological symptoms in dementia: A case report. *American Journal of Alzheimer's Disease & Other Dementias, 27,* 625–632.

Parker, G. B., Gayed, A., Owen, C. A., Hyett, M. P., Hilton, T. M., & Heruc, G. A. (2010). Survival following an acute coronary syndrome: A pet theory put to the test. *Acta Psychiatrica Scandinavica, 121,* 65–70.

Parslow, R. A., Jorm, A. F., Christensen, H., Rodgers, B., & Jacomb, P. (2005). Pet ownership and health in older adults: Findings from a survey of 2,551 community-based Australians aged 60–64. *Geronotology, 51,* 40–47.

Pedersen, B. K., & Saltin, B. (2006). Evidence for prescribing exercise as therapy in chronic disease. *Scandinavian Journal of Medicine and Science in Sports, 16*(S1), 3–63.

Pikhartova, J., Bowling, A., & Victor, C. (2014). Does owning a pet protect older people against loneliness? *BMC Geriatrics, 14,* 106. https://doi.org/10.1186/1471-2318-14-106.

Roberts, C. K., & Barnard, R. J. (2005). Effects of exercise and diet on chronic disease. *Journal of Applied Physiology, 98*(1), 3–30.

Rondeau, L., Corriveau, H., Bier, N., Camden, C., Champagne, N., & Dion, C. (2010). Effectiveness of a rehabilitation dog in fostering gait retraining for adults with a recent stroke: A multiple single-case study. *NeuroRehabilitation, 27,* 155–163.

Sellers, D. M. (2005). The evaluation of an animal assisted therapy intervention for elders with dementia in long-term care. *Activities, Adaptation, & Aging, 30,* 61–77.

Shibata, A., Oka, K., Inoue, S., Christian, H., Kitabatake, Y., & Shimomitsu, T. (2012). Physical activity of Japanese older adults who own and walk dogs. *American Journal of Preventive Medicine, 43,* 429–433.

Sloane, P. D., Zimmerman, S., Gruber-Baldini, A. L., & Barba, B. E. (2002). Plants, animals, and children in long-term care: How common are they? Do they affect clinical outcomes? *Alzheimer's Care Today, 3,* 12–18.

Stanley, I. H., Conwell, Y., Bowen, C., & Van Orden, K. A. (2014). Pet ownership may attenuate loneliness among older adult primary care patients who live alone. *Aging & Mental Health, 18,* 394–399.

Stasi, M., Amati, D., Costa, C., Resta, D., Senepa, G., Scarafioiti, C., & Molaschi, M. (2004). Pet-therapy: A trial for institutionalized frail elderly patients. *Archives of Gerontology and Geriatrics, 38,* 407–412.

Stewart, C. S., Thrush, J. C., Paulus, G. S., & Hafner, P. (1985). The elderly's adjustment to the loss of a companion animal: People–pet dependency. *Death Studies, 9,* 383–393.

Thorpe, R. J., Kreisle, R. A., Glickman, L. T., Simonsick, E. M., Newman, A. B., & Kritchevsky, S. (2006). Physical activity and pet ownership in year 3 of the health ABC study. *Journal of Aging and Physical Activity, 14,* 154–168.

Thorpe, R. J., Simonsick, E. M., Brach, J. S., Ayonayon, H., Satterfield, S., Harris, T. B., & Kritchevsky, S. B. (2006). Dog ownership, walking behavior, and maintained mobility in late life. *Journal of the American Geriatrics Society, 54,* 1419–1424.

Toohey, A. M., McCormack, G. R., Doyle-Baker, P. K., Adams, C. L., & Rock, M. J. (2013). Dog-walking and sense of community in neighborhoods: Implications for promoting regular physical activity in adults 50 years and older. *Health & Place, 22,* 75–81.

Travers, C., Perkins, J., Rand, J., Bartlett, H., & Morton, J. (2013). An evaluation of dog-assisted therapy for residents of aged care facilities with dementia. *Anthrozoös, 26,* 213–225.

U.S. Department of Health and Human Services. (2018). *Physical activity guidelines for Americans* (2nd ed.). Washington, DC: U.S. Department of Health and Human Services.

Vrbanac, Z., Zecevic, I., Ljubic, M., Belic, M., Stanin, D., Bottegaro, N. B., & Zubcic, D. (2013). Animal assisted therapy and perception of loneliness in geriatric nursing home residents. *Collegium Antropologicum, 37,* 973–976.

Walsh, P. G., Mertin, P. G., Verlander, D. F., & Pollard, C. F. (1995). The effects of a 'pets as therapy' dog on persons with dementia in a psychiatric ward. *Australian Occupational Therapy Journal, 42,* 161–166.

Wehofer, L., Goodson, N., & Shurtleff, T. L. (2013). Equine assisted activities and therapies: A case study of an older adult. *Physical & Occupational Therapy in Geriatrics, 31,* 71–87.

World Health Organization. (2011). *Information sheet: global recommendations on physical activity for health 65 years and above.* Retrieved from https://www.who.int/dietphysicalactivity/factsheet_olderadults/en/.

Winefield, H. R., Black, A., & Chur-Hansen, A. (2008). Health effects of ownership of and attachment to companion animals in an older population. *International Journal of Behavioral Medicine, 15,* 303–310.

Zisselman, M. H., Rovner, B. W., Shmuely, Y., & Ferrie, P. (1996). A pet therapy intervention with geriatric psychiatry inpatients. *American Journal of Occupational Therapy, 50,* 47–51.

**Nancy R. Gee, Ph.D.** is Professor of Psychiatry, Bill Balaban Chair of Human-Animal Interaction, and Director of the Center for Human-Animal Interaction in the School of Medicine at Virginia Commonwealth University. Previously Dr. Gee served as the Human-Animal Interaction Research Manager, for the Waltham Petcare Science Institute in Leicestershire England. She has published extensively on HAI, including her most recent book; *How Animals Help Students Learn: Research and Practice for Educators and Mental-Health Professionals.* Dr. Gee continues to pursue research in HAI across the lifespan, seeking to identify the ways in which interactions with companion animals affect human cognition, mental, and physical health. Concern for the animal's welfare and quality of life is a primary consideration for Dr. Gee, both in the Dogs on Call hospital visitation program she administers and in her various research and writing projects. Dr. Gee is a recipient of multiple grants and awards, a member of several organizational boards and journal editorial advisory boards, reviewer of HAI research grant proposals, and frequent presenter at national and international HAI conferences.

# Animal-Assisted Interactions Designed to Improve Human Wellbeing Across the Life Course

Nancy R. Gee

**Abstract** There is mounting evidence that interacting with a companion animal is beneficial to human health and well-being. Today's busy lifestyles involving working long hours or extensive travel can make it difficult for people to care for a companion animal, but there are now an increasing number and variety of programs involving animal interactions developed to benefit people of all ages. In this chapter we will discuss noteworthy examples that demonstrate the wide spectrum of Animal-Assisted Interaction (AAI) programs available. While a large number of these programs have not been scientifically tested or in many cases formally evaluated, we will discuss their intended and desired outcomes as well as the potential benefits that may arise from these sorts of interactions with companion animals. Additionally, we will include programs that represent a wide variety of animals from guinea pigs to horses and a wide variety of settings such as school and hospitals and court rooms.

**Keywords** Animal assisted therapy · Pet therapy · Stress reduction · Pets · Companion animals · Life course · Family life cycle · Child development · Caregiving · Stress · Aging · Health · Well-being · Bereavement · Human-animal interaction · Human-animal bond · Lifespan

Not everyone can have pets but, as the evidence related to the benefits of Human-Animal Interaction (HAI) accumulates, companion animals are being increasingly incorporated in a variety of unique and well-thought out interventions across a wide-range of settings with the intention of benefitting people of all ages. In this chapter we will discuss noteworthy examples of these Animal-Assisted Interactions (AAI) and the desired outcomes associated with the various activities and programs, but it is important to point out, that not all of these interactions have been explored scientifically, and our purpose in this chapter is not to present or evaluate a research evidence-base or even to comment on efficacy of these AAIs, but rather our intention

N. R. Gee (✉)
Center for Human-Animal Interaction, School of Medicine, Virginia Commonwealth University, Richmond, VA, USA
e-mail: Nancy.Gee@VCUHealth.org

is simply to describe the variety and potential benefits of the broad range of AAIs currently in use.

AAIs take many forms, some of which involve wild animals. This chapter will focus exclusively on interactions with animals that are typically kept as pets and considered companion animal species such as dogs, cats, and horses among others. AAI with wild animals, such as dolphins or Eagles, are controversial for a number of reasons, but not least of which is the stress to the animal of being required to live in captivity and be touched by, or come into close contact with humans, often to receive food.

It is important to consider the animal's perspective in these encounters, and to do so, we must have a good understanding the species needs and signs of stress in order to effectively evaluate their quality of life. Understanding their signs of stress is only the first step, we must also respect their needs and not require the animal to participate in an activity that is stressful or is demonstrably undesirable to the animal. It is important to give each animal a good life filled with safety, appropriate housing, nutrition and health care and activities they enjoy.

Now we will consider the wide-variety of AAIs implemented across the human life span and then we will return to the topic of the animal's perspective and quality of life at the end of this chapter. We will start our discussion with preschool age children, because there are currently no published reports of formalized AAI programs involving infants or toddlers.

## AAI and Preschoolers

By the time children reach preschool they are typically able to recognize and correctly identify common companion animals such as cats and kittens, dogs and puppies (Beck, 2011). Boys and girls both tend to be interested in, and demonstrate attachment to, animals. Anyone who has walked into a preschool classroom knows that animals are commonly depicted throughout the setting; on the walls, in books, in games and activities, and on children's clothes and shoes and backpacks. Teachers have long recognized children's interest in animals and use that interest to motivate learning, by including animals in lesson plans and bringing in classroom pets to teach children about empathy, animal welfare, and responsibility by learning to handle and care for animals.

Gee implemented a therapy dog-assisted preschool education program that involved twice weekly visits to an integrated preschool classroom that included typical and special needs preschool children ranging in age from 2 to 6 years. This program included one day of seated activities and one day of movement-based activities. In the seated activities, the children were asked to sit in a circle on a rug in their regular classroom and two therapy dogs were brought inside the circle separately, to provide lessons on specific topics. Each week, the children learned about a color, a number, and a shape. The dogs typically had the color on their collar, or vest, or on a toy they brought with them and the children were asked to find and identify the color of the week. Numbers were taught by asking the children to count with the dog who was prompted by hand signal to bark a specific number of times. Numbers were also taught be counting the dog's body parts. For example, the children might be asked how many ears does Louie have? Likewise, shapes were typically taught by asking the children to identify and name the shape of toys that the dog carried. When children were successful at naming a color, number, or shape, they were rewarded by getting to pet or brush the dog, or throw a toy to the dog to catch. Other lessons were incorporated about dogs and general dog care and varied from week to week. For example, the children were asked what dogs should eat (e.g., dog food) and what they shouldn't be allowed to eat (e.g., chocolate). Similarly, when the children got the answers right they received a dog-related reward as described above.

The movement-based activities took place in a large room with foam child flooring and specialized equipment that allowed the dogs and the children to use it, such as a large tunnel, jumps, and a balance beam. For this age group there is a connection between physical skill development and cognitive development (Rarick, 1980), so Gee wanted to capitalize on this connection by including the execution of gross motor skills in the program. These activities typically involved the dogs demonstrating a sequence of behaviors such as jump, walk across the balance beam, go through the tunnel and jump again. Once the children saw the sequence, they were asked to do the same sequence. On the next round the dog would demonstrate a different sequence. The dogs also "lead" games, stretching and relaxation activities. For example, in a game called "Louie Says" modeled after the popular "Simon Says" the handler would call out a behavior that the dog could do (e.g., sit, lay down, jump, prance) and either name the behavior or say "Louie says" and then name the behavior. If the children did the same behavior only after hearing "Louie says" they got it right and were able to continue in that round.

Following up on anecdotal reports of improvements in verbalizations, motor skills and social skills from parents and pre-school professionals as a result of this program Gee developed a series of a small-scale randomized control trials to evaluate the impact of the dogs' presence on aspects of behavior and cognition in preschool children. In one of these studies a mixed group of 14 typical and special needs (identified to have a language impairment) preschoolers participated in a motor skills task with a dog and with a human (Gee, Harris, & Johnson, 2007).

The children were evaluated on a series of skills designed to test locomotion, stability and manipulation. Depending on the task, they would either watch the dog perform and then mimic that behavior, or execute the behavior in tandem with the dog (in a short footrace, for instance). The results showed an increase in speed without a loss of accuracy when the dog was present, as compared with when the dog was absent.

In subsequent studies, Gee's laboratory assessed the effect of the presence or involvement of therapy dogs on motor and cognitive skills in preschoolers. They determined that preschoolers adhered to instructions better when modeling behaviors demonstrated by dogs (but not when competing, or acting in tandem, with the dogs) than by humans or stuffed dogs (Gee, Sherlock, Bennett, & Harris, 2009).

Similar positive results were found in a number of studies evaluating the cognitive impact of a dog's presence directly. For instance, while performing a memory task, preschoolers required fewer instructional prompts when a dog was present than in the presence of a stuffed dog or a human (Gee, Crist, & Carr, 2010).

At around the same time the Gee program was running Kotrschal and Ortbauer (2003) reported on the behavioral effects of having a dog in a classroom of children (average age 6.7 years) in Vienna, Austria. In this study, the researchers were able to video tape the classroom activities before the dog joined and then systematically while the dog was present in the classroom. They used an objective scoring method to examine specific child behaviors before and during the presence of the dog. Kotrschal and Ortbauer found that the children became more socially integrated when the dog was present, and that this effect was more pronounced for boys than for girls. Even though the children spent a lot of time watching the dog, they also paid more attention to the teacher. The researchers concluded that the presence of a dog in a classroom positively stimulates social cohesion and provides a reasonably inexpensive means of improving the learning environment.

## AAI and Primary School Age Children

In recent decades researchers have explored the potential benefits of animal interventions in two key elements of child development: reading, an essential component of learning and life success, and social skills.

### *AAI and Reading/Cognition*

Much has been written about the potential for dogs to improve children's reading skills. The seminal program, R.E.A.D.®, Reading Education Assistance Dogs®, was begun by Intermountain Therapy Animals in 1999; over 6,000 therapy animal teams have trained and registered with this program, with affiliated programs in the U.S., Canada, Mexico and 24 other countries around the world (therapyanimals.org). Other organizations run similar programs. Although research to substantiate these claims is sparse, and the underlying mechanisms are unclear (Hall, Gee, & Mills, 2016), the children, teachers, parents and therapy teams involved believe the programs to be effective and at least random control one study (Le Roux, Swartz, & Swart, 2014) found evidence in favor of such programs.

In programs such as R.E.A.D.®, a child practices reading aloud to a dog, with the dog's handler present to insure everyone's safety, though typically not directly participating in the reading process. Because the dog is perceived as non-judgmental, the child can relax and learn to enjoy reading in a non-stressful environment, thus making quicker progress in skill development than otherwise. Another approach, more common in Europe than in the United States, has a classroom dog present while a teacher, often the dog's owner, works with children on conventional reading education strategies. The dog's presence is considered to add a relaxing and fun element to the learning process.

Among the suggested theories underlying the effectiveness of any program involving dogs and reading are motivation (the possibility that the dog triggers an intrinsic motivation), a sense of security triggered by the dogs and traceable to the biophilia hypothesis, and an increased oxytocin (and corresponding decrease in stress) release tied to the presence of the dog (Beetz & McCardle, 2017). While dogs cannot teach children to read without prior intervention in the basics by a teacher or parent, it appears that their presence may enhance the abilities of those who already have the basic skills in place.

As noted above, research has found enhanced cognitive functioning in preschoolers in the presence of dogs (Gee et al., 2009; Gee, Belcher, Grabski, DeJesus, & Riley, 2012; Gee, Church, & Altobelli, 2010; Gee, Crist, & Carr, 2010; Gee, Gould, Swanson, & Wagner, 2012). A 2019 study by Brelsford, et al. found similar results when a group of 8–9 year olds were evaluated on the performance of a Stroop test after spending unstructured time with a dog as compared with an equivalent amount of time spend in meditation (Brelsford, Meints, & Gee, Under Review). Success in a Stroop test, which measures an individual's ability to override the automatic process of reading to name a color. For example, they may be presented with the word "blue" written in red ink. Their task is to name the color of ink (red), but to do that they have to override the automatic process of reading (quick response of saying "blue"). Performance on this task benefits from greater concentration and less haste in responding. The results of this study suggest improved executive functioning on the part of the students who interacted with the dogs. Executive functioning is a cluster of processes, including the ability to inhibit quick, but often erroneous responses. Higher levels of executive functioning have been associated with academic and life success (Hediger, Gee, & Griffin, 2017). The results of this study indicate that executive functioning can be improved by interacting with a dog.

## *AAI and Social Behavior Deficits*

The social skills and behaviors of children affect their educational success and their ability to function in the real world, as well as the students and teachers with whom they share classrooms. There is evidence to suggest that the presence of animals in a classroom can help in this regard. As discussed previously, the Kortrschal and Ortbauer (2003) study demonstrated that a dog's presence in a classroom of 6-year-olds could contribute to social cohesion and improved teaching conditions.

Another study with a similar finding involved a larger group of primary school age children, 64 in the experimental group and 64 in a wait-listed control group (O'Haire, McKenzie, McCune, & Slaughter, 2013). The children in the experimental group were given an introductory lesson about guinea pigs, covering both their food and housing needs and appropriate handling. That was followed by twice-weekly open interactions with the 2 guinea pigs who lived in the classroom during the study. During these 20-min sessions the children engaged in a wide range of guinea pig-related activities, including feeding, grooming, toy making, health monitoring, and unstructured interactions. The experimental group were found by both teachers and parents to have greater increases in social skills and decreases in problem behaviors than the control group. Once again, the conclusion of the researchers was that the animal assisted interventions could improve social functioning in a classroom of young children.

Pendry and colleagues have found improvements in various aspects of children's social competence in a non-classroom, after-school equine therapy experiment (Pendry, Carr, Smith, & Roeter, 2014). Participants, not all of whom began the experiment suffering shortcomings in social skills, spent time in the presence of the horses over the course of the 11-week program. The children began by learning about safety, horse behavior and herd dynamics, then moved on to moving horses through gentle pressure, leading them and reading their body language, driving them forward through body language, riding them, desensitizing them, massaging them, demonstrating riding skills learned, and "teaching" others about horses. Through these exercises the children improved their skills with regard to respect, communication, leadership, trust, boundaries, overcoming challenges, and self regulation.

At the conclusion of the study positive behaviors had increased and negative behaviors had decreased for the participants, with greater changes tied to more regular attendance in the program. Pendry et al. took pains to note that these benefits likely derived not just from interacting with the horses, but from the structure of the program.

## *AAI and Psychotherapy for Children*

In the mid-1960s child psychologist Dr. Boris Levison realized that when his dog was present, therapy sessions with children were often more productive, with the patients more willing to communicate. Although his initial presentation of these observations was met with derision, opinions began to change when it emerged that Sigmund Freud had noted the same phenomenon with his own dog (Coren, 2010). Fifty years later animal assisted therapy (AAT) is widespread.

Simply arranging for a companion animal to be present in a therapy session does not predetermine success. The therapist must evaluate for each patient whether the animal may indeed be a helpful adjunct to a traditional treatment approach, and if so, the specific the animal-based intervention to take.

Aubrey Fine, well known for involving a variety of animals in his own child psychotherapy practice, and tireless advocate for the adoption of best practices in the field, provides clinical examples in support of a range of theories as to the mechanism behind the effectiveness AAT in Handbook on Animal-Assisted Therapy: Theoretical Foundations and Guidelines for Practice.

<u>Animals can be a social lubricant to initiate therapy</u>, when the desire to interact with the animal encourages previously non-communicative children to open up. <u>Animals can act as a bridge to establish a relationship with the therapist</u>, as when discussions of a shared interest in a specific animal or a type of animal can introduce therapeutic opportunities. <u>Animals may serve as an emotional trigger</u>; the presence

of an animal can break down inhibitions that may otherwise exist between a child and a therapist, allowing those emotions to be addressed, and an animal, particularly one that is furry or cuddly, can provide a type of physical support that would be inappropriate if administered by the therapist. <u>Animals can model appropriate behaviors,</u> in the form of either restraint or enthusiasm, or as in a particularly poignant example cited by Fine, the right to establish boundaries for physical touch (Fine, 2019).

Often the animals involved in psychotherapy sessions have been selected, trained and owned by the therapist. Given the sensitive circumstances it is essential that the animal is comfortable with—and even enjoys—being part of the therapy team. Although golden retrievers are often cited as having an almost natural affinity for this work, not every dog in the breed is equally well suited to offering support and absorbing and dissipating the emotional output of the patients. Animals who are part of therapy teams can suffer "burnout" from their intense roles, and the need to limit the frequency and duration of their participation must be respected.

In some circumstances the therapy animal may have a separate owner/trainer/handler who is present during AAT. These situations may lack the intimacy of the three-way interventions (patient-animal-therapist) but may offer benefits otherwise not available, if, for instance, the intervention must occur outside the therapist's office, or if large animals such as horses are involved and safety is a concern. In the Canine Advocates program described below, the dogs' handlers wear noise-cancelling headphones to preserve the confidentiality of the patient-therapist relationship.

## *AAI and Trauma Counseling for Children*

A particularly striking example of how a highly trained therapy dog can help children work through trauma is the Canine Advocates program within the Center for Victims in Pittsburgh, Pennsylvania. Over 100 specifically trained facility dogs work in courthouses in three dozen states, helping children and vulnerable adults feel less stressed and more secure when offering testimony. At times, less rigorously trained therapy dogs are permitted to provide the same service, although the use of any dogs in the witness box is not without controversy. Some attorneys argue that the presence of the dog biases juries against defendants, although others claim that victims or witnesses who cry or shut down on the stand are even more prejudicial (Bergal, 2017).

What is unique about the Canine Advocates program is that this small, carefully selected and trained group of dogs works with child victims throughout the entire post-trauma process, not just in the courtroom (T. Potts, personal communication, November 6, 2019). They are present from forensic interview to medical exam, in therapy visits, district attorney meetings, and courtroom testimony. This ongoing relationship allows the development of a bond between the child and the dog, providing a greater level of comfort and a potential boost to healing that would not otherwise be present. Although a program such as this is not adaptable to controlled testing, other evidence indicates that the effectiveness of Animal Assisted Interventions is more pronounced when a bond exists between the human and the animal—or even if the human has a positive history of pet ownership.

## AAI and Young Adults

It is no secret that U.S. college students today report much higher levels of stress than previous generations. The litany of stressors goes beyond the struggle to achieve academic success, or even to get into the courses they need in their chosen field. It includes direct physical fears such as mass shootings or sexual assault; concerns over the future of the nation and the world in the face of climate change, immigration and deportations; and crushing student debt and the decreasing value of the wages they can earn upon graduation (McClennen, 2019).

While these troublesome feelings can exist throughout the semester/trimester/school year, they often come to a head at exam time, when stress and anxiety, regardless of their cause, can interfere with effective studying test-taking. As a countermeasure, over 900 Animal Visitation Programs ("AVPs"), typically running concurrent with or just prior to "exam week", have been initiated in colleges and universities across the U.S. and Canada (Crossman & Kazdin, 2015). These programs are not therapy sessions, but rather opportunities for individuals to interact with animals for brief periods with the goal of temporary stress reduction. They are efficient and flexible, often occurring in group sessions in libraries or similar facilities, and they lack the potential stigma attached to visits to counseling centers.

Perhaps most importantly, the student participants go into the interactions with the assumption that they will be helpful. And indeed, based on participant perceptions (though not physiological measures), AVPs can produce an increase in positive mood and a reduction in anxiety and negative mood on a short-term or moment-to-moment basis when compared with control conditions (Barker, Barker, McCain, & Schubert, 2016; Crossman, Kazdin, & Knudson, 2015; Pendry, Carr, Roeter, & Vandagriff, 2018).

A more intensive approach has been examined in a 4-week randomized control trial during which they compared three conditions: evidence based academic stress management counseling, human-animal interactions only, and a combination of the two (Pendry, Kuzara, & Gee, 2019). The student participants in this study found the combination approach, where dogs were present during the presentation of the evidence-based content, to be the most effective. In the words of the study authors, "The presence and engagement with animals appeared to serve as a momentary source of relaxation as well as a motivator for involvement with content, which may enhance adaptation of student adaptive stress management techniques and coping for long term advantage" (p. 11).

## AAI and Special Populations of Children

Along with their investigation of the effects of AAI involving guinea pigs on the social behaviors of school children described above, O'Haire et al. also explored the effects of the guinea pigs on children with autism spectrum disorder (ASD) (O'Haire, McKenzie, Beck, & Slaughter, 2013). Specifically, the researchers evaluated the interactions of children with ASD with adults and with other, typically developing, children, when they were allowed to play with guinea pigs as compared with playing with toys. In the presence of the guinea pigs the children with ASD demonstrated significantly more pro-social behaviors toward the other humans, and showed warmth and affection to the animals (though not the humans).

In looking at the potential reasons for these improvements, the O'Haire et al. team found that the guinea pigs may serve as social buffers. When comparing the levels of physiological arousal of children with ASD across four different activities, this measure of stress was higher than that of traditionally developing children in all cases except when interacting with the guinea pigs. The animals seem to have reduced the ASD children's stress levels (O'Haire, McKenzie, Beck, & Slaughter, 2015).

While guinea pigs have proved to be excellent choices for testing the effects of animals on children with ASD, in general dogs are the most common animal working with this population. Although they are not ideal (a dog's smell or barking may be problematic), their natural behaviors as well as their non-judgmental nature can be appealing to children with ASD, reducing negative and increasing positive behaviors. To a lesser extent, equine assisted therapy, particularly in the form of Therapeutic Horseback Riding (THR) has been found to be helpful, whether because of the rhythmic movement of the horse or other reasons (Grandin, Fine, O'Haire, Carlisle, & Bowers, 2019).

Another intellectual developmental disorder that seemingly responds to AAI is attention deficit hyperactivity disorder (ADHD). In a 12-week randomized trial that added canine assisted interventions (CAI) to traditional cognitive behavioral group therapy for children identified with ADHD, those children receiving the CAI demonstrated greater declines in ADHD symptoms than the control group (Schuck et al., 2018). As part of the Positive Assertive Cooperative Kids (P.A.C.K.) curriculum employed in this study, the children learned to "train" basic commands such as sit and stay to certified therapy dogs. Counselors taught children how to read and appropriately respond to dogs' nonverbal behavior, as well as the skills, such as remaining calm, necessary to successfully interact with the dogs. Even the social skill development elements of the P.A.C.K. curriculum that did not involve direct interactions with dogs included dog related themes (Schuck, Fine, Abdullah, & Lakes, 2019).

## AAI and Special Populations of Adults

Although animals can be included in adult psychotherapy sessions in many of the same ways as with children's counseling, AAI programs for adults in special populations are rapidly growing. The Canine Advocates program referenced above, for instance, is available to vulnerable adults as well as to children.

## *AAI and the US Military Personnel*

The press surrounding efforts to convince the US Veterans Administration to approve service dogs as a treatment for post traumatic stress disorder ("PTSD") has overshadowed the longstanding connections between dogs (and other animals) and the US military healthcare system. In 1919, following World War I, canine therapeutic interventions were used with psychiatric patients at St. Elizabeth's Hospital in Washington, DC (Velde, Cipriani, & Fisher, 2005). During World War II, resident farm animals were integrated into treatment programs at the Army Airforce Convalescent Center in Pawling, NY, a facility where veterans recuperated from combat related emotional fatigue (Chumley, 2012).

Today, AAA and AAT programs are incorporated in military hospitals around the country. Animal assisted activities in VA hospitals are similar to those in non-military medical facilities, typically taking the form of either group meetings in common areas, or individual visits by the animals and handlers in patient rooms. Military hospitals also use volunteer animals as part of goal directed physical, occupational, recreational, speech-language or other rehabilitation therapy programs (Veterans Health Administration, 2018). In October 2019, the Veterans Administration announced a collaboration with Pet Partners Inc., a leading provider of animal assisted interventions, to extend their offerings (US Dept of Veterans Affairs press release dated November 7, 2019).

Since 2007, a rotating series of dogs have been incorporated into the US Army's Combat Operational Stress Control ("COSC") programs in Iraq and Afghanistan (Smith-Forbes, Najera, & Hawkins, 2014). Along with being general morale boosters, the dogs served as social lubricants, allowing the occupational therapists to form connections with soldiers quickly, circumventing the stigma that is often attached to accepting offers of assistance with mental health issues (Fike, Najera, & Dougherty, 2012). Only dogs who make it through rigorous training programs designed to test social skills in stressful environments and tolerance to extreme weather and noise conditions are accepted into the program (Krol, 2012). Upon completion of their deployment, COSC dogs are offered their own rehabilitation time if they appear to be suffering compassion fatigue, and then redeployed, often to occupational or physical therapy programs at military bases (Kaplan, 2015).

A highly successful AAT initiative now available at many military basis and hospitals is the Warrior Canine Connection's (WCC's) Mission Based Trauma Recovery

(MBTR) program (Yount, Koffman, & Olmert, 2019). MBTR participants are trained to be dog trainers, a process that can reduce PTSD symptoms (Yount, Olmert, & Lee, 2012) and teach skills that the soldiers can use as they transition to civilian life (Tedeschi, Sisa, Olmert, Parish-Plass, & Yount, 2015). "Bonding with and shaping the behavior of young dogs offer unlimited experiential training opportunities for wounded warriors to practice patience, empathy, and consistency" (pp. 359–360). The MBTR is not a stand-alone therapy, but used in conjunction with conventional PTSD treatment modalities.

A preliminary study by Krause-Parello et al. of the effects on veterans suffering from PTSD of walking shelter dogs as compared with walking alongside a human along the same route suggested that benefits accrued from the experience for those veterans with the greatest existing PTSD indicators (Krause-Parello, Friedmann, Blanchard, Payton, & Gee, 2020). Additional studies evaluating higher dosages (i.e. more walks per week or more weeks of walking) along with modifications to the study design may provide more meaningful results.

## *Equine AAI and Abused Adult Women*

It has been speculated that because the horse is a prey animal it is more sensitive to minute changes in human's emotional state. Additionally, unique interactions are possible with a horse, since it is able to bear the weight of a human (Latella & Abrams, 2019). Equine therapy has been found useful for women struggling to overcome abuse and trauma and attempting to rebuild their lives, by allowing them to enrich their skills and their self-confidence (Froeschle, 2009). In a qualitative study of five women who had suffered abuse, equine facilitated psychotherapy was found to be an effective intervention (Meinersmann, Bradberry, & Roberts, 2008). The elements of an equine therapy program for victims of abuse can be complex, and the mechanisms can be unclear, but the results have often been found to be beneficial (Shambo, Seely, & Vonderfecht, 2010).

## AAI and Older Adults

As noted in chapter "Successful Aging and Human-Animal Interaction", pet ownership declines with age, but that does not necessarily mean that older adults no longer enjoy spending time with companion animals. They may lack the funds or the physical ability to care for a pet, or they have changed housing circumstances that prohibit pets. Animal assisted interventions can help them stay connected with the animal world.

In some cases, the intervenor can actually be human, providing services or funds to allow older adults to keep their pets in their homes. Organizations exist in nearly every state that help pay for veterinary care. The Senior Pet Assistance Network, a 503(c) charity in Dallas, Texas is a shining example of a community working together to help keep older adults and their companion animals together (Senior Pets Assistance Network, 2019). Meals on Wheels America has had a pet assistance program since 2007, which has been supported since 2015 by Banfield Charitable Trust and Petsmart, allowing them to deliver pet food, grooming, veterinary visits and other support to older pet owners through over 360 local Meals on Wheels programs (Meals on Wheels America, 2019).

There are also organizations such as Pet Peace of Mind that help older adults who need hospice care (Pet Peace of Mind, 2018). In the words of Pet Peace of Mind president Diane McGill, "I know of countless patients who have said that their pet is their lifeline. Pets are great medicine for coping with the anxiety the comes from dealing with a serious medical condition. For many patients, keeping their pets near them during the end of life journey and finding homes for their beloved pets after they pass is one of the most important pieces of unfinished business" (Pet Peace of Mind, 2018, About Us, Paragraph 5). Pet Peace of Mind volunteers routinely tend to all pet care chores, and if the owner must transfer to a health care facility, they arrange for the pet to be boarded, and eventually, adopted.

When relocation to a long-term residential facility is unavoidable, older adults can still enjoy animal companionship through facility animals or visits from volunteers who bring in their own pets, typically dogs. Usually these volunteer teams are affiliated with national or local therapy animal registries such as Pet Partners, Inc. or Therapy Dogs International, which provide training, vetting and insurance. Time spent with these visitors can be quiet, with the older adult simply petting or cuddling with the animal, or can be more active, as when the residents take the dogs for a walk.

## AAI in Acute Care Hospital Settings

Individuals of all ages may encounter AAI during hospital stays. Although some institutions will allow visits by patients' own pets, a potential stress alleviator and mood booster, more typically AAI in hospitals occurs in the form of visits by certified therapy dog teams.

Dogs On Call ("DOC") is a popular therapy dog program established by the Virginia Commonwealth University ("VCU") School of Medicine—Center For Human Animal Interaction in 2001. During their stay, patients at any of VCU hospitals and treatment centers have the opportunity to be visited by one of the 90+ DOC therapy dog teams. The DOC program guidelines for dog-and-handler team training and health screening, as well as other safety considerations for both patients and dogs, have been documented in detail by program founder Sandra Barker (Barker, Vokes, & Barker, 2019).

## Conclusion

The examples of AAI provided in this chapter vary considerably, yet this list is not exhaustive. Given our long, shared history of companionship with animals, particularly dogs, it isn't surprising to see the many variants on AAI that people have concocted. It is clear that the human-animal bond is seen as a valuable mechanism for treating, improving, or otherwise positively impacting the lives of people across the developmental spectrum and those individuals in a wide variety of special populations and circumstances.

Generally, there is something of a common-sense acceptance of the positive effects of interacting with animals. Some examples include the notions that interacting with animals reduces loneliness, depression, stress and anxiety, and improves mood, life expectancy, and quality of life. People tend to see companion animals as being beneficial to humans for a number of reasons, whether those reasons are backed by scientific evidence or not, is often irrelevant.

Because AAIs tend to be low cost, low risk and very popular with recipients, there is little reason for the uninitiated not to implement them. However, relying on a scientifically established evidence-base will allow for the implementation of the most safe and effective AAIs. Furthermore, it is critical to have a complete understanding of the needs of the species involved and as part of an implementation protocol to establish clear procedures to care for the health and well-being of the animals involved. To be very clear, it is not enough to stop there. An ethically implemented AAI will include an evaluation of the AAI protocols and specifically the role of the animals, by a disinterested third party. For instance, the infection prevention and control protocols established for the Dogs on Call program at the Virginia Commonwealth University (Barker et al., 2019) were reviewed by the Society for Healthcare Epidemiology of America, which has prepared AAI best practice recommendations for hospitals and other acute care facilities (Murthy et al., 2015).

This chapter presents some examples of the wide variety of AAIs that are currently in use in the United States, and around the world. As you can see, there is good reason to be excited about the future of these sorts of programs, but we shouldn't lose track of the need to evaluate their implementation and efficacy simply because they tend to be fun, and low cost and low risk. It is of critical importance to put people and pets together in situations that are truly safe, effective, and beneficial for all involved.

## References

Barker, S. B., Barker, R. T., McCain, N. L., & Schubert, C. M. (2016). A randomized cross-over exploratory study of the effect of visiting therapy dogs on college student stress before final exams. *Anthrozoös, 29*(1), 35–46.

Barker, S. B., Vokes, R. A., & Barker, R. T. (2019). *Animal-assisted interventions in health care settings: A best practices manual for establishing new programs (New directions in the human-animal bond)*. West Lafayette: Purdue University Press.

Beck, A. M. (2011). Animals and child health and development. *Animals in our lives: Human-animal interaction in family, community, and therapeutic settings*, 43–52.

Beetz, A., & McCardle, P. (2017). Does reading to a dog affect reading skills. *How animals help students learn: Research and practice for educators and mental health professionals*, 111–123.

Bergal, J. (2017). *Canines helping out in the courtroom*. Retrieved November 6, 2019, from https://www.pewtrusts.org/en/research-and-analysis/blogs/stateline/2017/06/26/canines-helping-out-in-the-courtroom.

Brelsford, V., Meints, K., & Gee, N. R. (Under Review). Effects of animal-assisted interventions on executive functioning in school children. *International Journal of Environmental Research and Public Health*.

Chumley, P. R. (2012). Historical perspectives of the human-animal bond within the Department of Defense. *US Army Medical Department Journal*, 18–21.

Coren, S. (2010). Foreword. *Handbook on Animal-Assisted Therapy*. (pp. xxv–xxvi). San Diego: Academic Press.

Crossman, M. K., & Kazdin, A. E. (2015). Animal visitation programs in colleges and universities: An efficient model for reducing student stress. In *Handbook on animal-assisted therapy* (pp. 333–337). San Diego: Academic Press.

Crossman, M. K., Kazdin, A. E., & Knudson, K. (2015). Brief unstructured interaction with a dog reduces distress. *Anthrozoös, 28*(4), 649–659.

Fike, L., Najera, C., & Dougherty, D. (2012). Occupational therapists as dog handlers: the collective experience with animal-assisted therapy in Iraq. *US Army Medical Department Journal*.

Fine, A. H. (2019). Best practices in animal-assisted therapy: Guidelines for use of AAT with special populations. In *Handbook on animal-assisted therapy* (pp. 207–224). San Diego: Academic Press.

Froeschle, J. (2009). Empowering abused women through equine assisted career therapy. *Journal of Creativity in Mental Health, 4*(2), 180–190.

Gee, N. R., Belcher, J., Grabski, J., DeJesus, M., & Riley, W. (2012). The presence of a therapy dog results in improved object recognition performance in preschool children. *Anthrozoös, 25*, 289–300.

Gee, N. R., Church, M. T., & Altobelli, C. L. (2010). Preschoolers make fewer errors on an object categorization task in the presence of a dog. *Anthrozoös, 23*, 223–230.

Gee, N. R., Crist, E. N., & Carr, D. N. (2010). Preschool children require fewer instructional prompts to perform a memory task in the presence of a dog. *Anthrozoös, 23*, 178–184.

Gee, N. R., Gould, J. K., Swanson, C. C., & Wagner, A. K. (2012). Preschoolers categorize animate objects better in the presence of a dog. *Anthrozoös, 25*, 187–198.

Gee, N. R., Harris, S. L., & Johnson, K. L. (2007). The role of therapy dogs in speed and accuracy to complete motor skills tasks for preschool children. *Anthrozoös, 20*, 375–386.

Gee, N. R., Sherlock, T. R., Bennett, E. A., & Harris, S. L. (2009). Preschoolers' adherence to instructions as a function of the presence of a dog, and motor skills task. *Anthrozoös, 22*, 267–276.

Grandin, T., Fine, A. H., O'Haire, M. E., Carlisle, G., & Bowers, C. M. (2019). The roles of animals for individuals with autism spectrum disorder. In *Handbook on animal-assisted therapy* (pp. 285–298). San Diego: Academic Press.

Hall, S. S., Gee, N. R., & Mills, D. S. (2016). Children reading to dogs: A systematic review of the literature. *PLoS ONE, 11*(2), e0149759.

Hediger, K., Gee, N. R., & Griffin, J. A. (2017) Do animal in the classroom improve learning, attention, or other aspects of cognition. In N. R. Gee & A. H. Fine (Eds.), *How animals help students learn: Research and practice for educators and mental-health professionals* (pp. 56–68). Routledge Taylor & Francis Group.

Intermountain Therapy Animals. (2018). *Intermountain therapy animals: About us*. Retrieved November 6, 2019 from http://www.therapyanimals.org/Contact_Us.html.

Kaplan, M. D. (2015). *Dogs bring relief to soldiers operation stress control*. Retrieved November 12, 2019 from https://thebark.com/content/dogs-bring-relief-soldiers.

Kotrschal, K., & Ortbauer, B. (2003). Behavioral effects of the presence of a dog in a classroom. *Anthrozoös, 16*(2), 147–159.

Krause-Parello, C. A., Friedmann, E., Blanchard, K., Payton, M., & Gee, N. R. (2020). Veterans and shelter dogs: Examining the impact of a dog-walking intervention on physiological and post-traumatic stress symptoms. *Anthrozoös, 33*(2), 225–241.

Krol, W. (2012). Training the combat and operational stress control dog: An innovative modality for behavioral health. *US Army Medical Department Journal.*

Latella, D., & Abrams, B. N. (2019). The role of the equine in animal-assisted interactions. In *Handbook on animal-assisted therapy* (pp. 133–162). San Diego: Academic Press.

Le Roux, M. C., Swartz, L., & Swart, E. (2014, December). The effect of an animal-assisted reading program on the reading rate, accuracy and comprehension of grade 3 students: A randomized control study. In *Child & Youth Care Forum* (Vol. 43, No. 6, pp. 655–673). Springer US.

McClennen, S. (2019, September 15). *Why are college students so stressed out? It's not because they're "snowflakes".* Retrieved November 27, 2019 from https://www.salon.com/2019/09/15/why-are-college-students-so-stressed-out-its-not-because-theyre-snowflakes/.

Meals on Wheels America. (2019). *Keeping seniors and their pets together.* Retrieved November 27, 2019, from https://www.mealsonwheelsamerica.org/take-action/senior-pet-support.

Meinersmann, K. M., Bradberry, J., & Roberts, F. B. (2008). Equine-facilitated psychotherapy with adult female survivors of abuse. *Journal of Psychosocial Nursing and Mental Health Services, 46*(12), 36–42.

Murthy, R., Bearman, G., Brown, S., Bryant, K., Chinn, R., Hewlett, A., … Wiemken, T. (2015). Animals in healthcare facilities: Recommendations to minimize potential risks. *Infection Control & Hospital Epidemiology, 36*(5), 495–516.

O'Haire, M. E., McKenzie, S. J., Beck, A. M., & Slaughter, V. (2013). Social behaviors increase in children with autism in the presence of animals compared to toys. *PLoS ONE, 8*(2), e57010.

O'Haire, M. E., McKenzie, S. J., Beck, A. M., & Slaughter, V. (2015). Animals may act as social buffers: Skin conductance arousal in children with autism spectrum disorder in a social context. *Developmental Psychobiology, 57*(5), 584–595.

O'Haire, M. E., McKenzie, S. J., McCune, S., & Slaughter, V. (2013). Effects of animal-assisted activities with guinea pigs in the primary school classroom. *Anthrozoös, 26*(3), 445–458.

Pendry, P., Carr, A. M., Roeter, S. M., & Vandagriff, J. L. (2018). Experimental trial demonstrates effects of animal-assisted stress prevention program on college students' positive and negative emotion. *Human-Animal Interaction Bulletin, 6*(1), 81–97.

Pendry, P., Carr, A. M., Smith, A. N., & Roeter, S. M. (2014). Improving adolescent social competence and behavior: A randomized trial of an 11-week equine facilitated learning prevention program. *The Journal of Primary Prevention, 35*(4), 281–293.

Pendry, P., Kuzara, S., & Gee, N. R. (2019). Evaluation of undergraduate students' responsiveness to a 4-week university-based animal-assisted stress prevention program. *International Journal of Environmental Research and Public Health, 16*(18), 3331.

Pet Peace of Mind. (2018). *Pet peace of mind helps hospice and seriously ill patients keep their pets.* Retrieved November 27, 2019, from https://petpeaceofmind.org/about-us/.

Rarick, G. L. (1980). Cognitive-motor relationships in the growing years. *Research Quarterly for Exercise and Sport, 51*(1), 174–192.

Schuck, S. E. B., Fine, A. H., Abdullah, M. M., & Lakes, K. D. (2019). Animal assisted interventions for children with disorders of executive function: The influence of humane education and character development on the P.A.C.K. model. In *Handbook on animal-assisted therapy* (pp. 115–137). San Diego: Academic Press.

Schuck, S. E., Johnson, H. L., Abdullah, M. M., Stehli, A., Fine, A. H., & Lakes, K. D. (2018). The role of animal assisted intervention on improving self-esteem in children with attention deficit/hyperactivity disorder. *Frontiers in Pediatrics, 6,* 300.

Senior Pet Assistance Network. (2019). *About Us.* Retrieved November 12, 2019, from https://www.seniorspets.org/aboutus.htm.

Shambo, L., Seely, S. K., & Vonderfecht, H. (2010). A pilot study on equine-facilitated psychotherapy for trauma-related disorders. *Scientific and Educational Journal of Therapeutic Riding, 16,* 11–23.

Smith-Forbes, E., Najera, C., & Hawkins, D. (2014). Combat operational stress control in Iraq and Afghanistan: Army occupational therapy. *Military Medicine, 179*(3), 279–284.

Tedeschi, P., Sisa, M. L., Olmert, M. D., Parish-Plass, N., & Yount, R. (2015). Treating human trauma with the help of animals: trauma informed intervention for child maltreatment and adult post-traumatic stress. In *Handbook on animal-assisted therapy* (pp. 363–380). San Diego: Academic Press.

Velde, B. P., Cipriani, J., & Fisher, G. (2005). Resident and therapist views of animal-assisted therapy: Implications for occupational therapy practice. *Australian Occupational Therapy Journal, 52*(1), 43–50.

Veterans Health Administration. (2018). *Animal-Assisted Activities and Animal-Assisted Therapy* (VHA Directive 1178(1)). U.S. Department of Veterans Affairs.

Yount, R. A., Koffman, R., & Olmert, M. D. (2019). The battle for hearts and minds: Warrior canine connection's mission-based trauma recovery program. *New Directions In The Human-Animal Bond*, 355.

Yount, R. A., Olmert, M. D., & Lee, M. R. (2012). Service dog training program for treatment of posttraumatic stress in service members. *US Army Medical Department Journal*.

**Nancy R. Gee, Ph.D.** is Professor of Psychiatry, Bill Balaban Chair of Human-Animal Interaction, and Director of the Center for Human-Animal Interaction in the School of Medicine at Virginia Commonwealth University. Previously Dr. Gee served as the Human-Animal Interaction Research Manager, for the Waltham Petcare Science Institute in Leicestershire England. She has published extensively on HAI, including her most recent book; *How Animals Help Students Learn: Research and Practice for Educators and Mental-Health Professionals.* Dr. Gee continues to pursue research in HAI across the lifespan, seeking to identify the ways in which interactions with companion animals affect human cognition, mental, and physical health. Concern for the animal's welfare and quality of life is a primary consideration for Dr. Gee, both in the Dogs on Call hospital visitation program she administers and in her various research and writing projects. Dr. Gee is a recipient of multiple grants and awards, a member of several organizational boards and journal editorial advisory boards, reviewer of HAI research grant proposals, and frequent presenter at national and international HAI conferences.

# Conclusion

Nancy R. Gee

**Abstract** We have provided a brief overview of the many ways that Human-Animal Interaction may impact human well-being over the life course. In so doing we have highlighted a number of key topics and discussed the merits of the relevant evidence, but there remain a few important topics to consider. For example, there is evidence to indicate that our relationships with companion animals have changed substantially in recent years suggesting that in this concluding chapter it is critical to discuss the larger, societal perspective. We must consider the needs of the animal and provide a better understanding of the challenges related to studying pet ownership as a variable in research. And, finally, we conclude with specific recommendations to guide future research.

**Keywords** Animal assisted therapy · Pet therapy · Stress reduction · Pets · Companion animals · Life course · Family life cycle · Child development · Caregiving · Stress · Aging · Health · Well-being · Bereavement · Human-animal interaction · Human-animal bond · Lifespan

In this brief exploration of how Human-Animal Interaction (HAI) may impact human well-being over the life course we have highlighted a number of key topics, but there remain a few gaps in our overall discussion that we aim to fill in this concluding chapter. The impact of HAI on human health and well-being is wide-ranging, and although we have discussed this issue from many angles and even across the developmental life span, here we take a step back and examine human-animal interaction at the societal and cultural levels.

To accomplish this goal, we should start with the evidence indicating that the very nature of human-animal relationships has changed substantially in recent years (Fox & Gee, 2016). In the past 30 years for example, we have seen a rapid change in attitudes and practices concerning companion animals. Examples include advances

---

N. R. Gee (✉)
Center for Human-Animal Interaction, School of Medicine, Virginia Commonwealth University, Richmond, VA, USA
e-mail: Nancy.Gee@VCUHealth.org

in veterinary medicine and pet nutrition, improved understanding of animal behavior and needs, and even transformation of the very places animals live within our homes and families. Companion animals are increasingly humanized, reflected in a rapid increase in companion animal populations at the same time they are being increasingly integrated into the home and family. Animals use to serve a function, such a herding livestock, and they frequently lived in barns or dog houses. Now they most frequently live inside the home, tend to be considered members of the family, and are not required to serve any function beyond that of companionship. In some cases, attachment to pets has gone to the extreme. Some pet owners dress their pets up routinely or carry them around in handbags, and these or others may profess an inability to function without their pet's emotional support.

Pet commercialization has mushroomed in recent decades (Fox & Gee, 2016) with consumers now having ready access to personalized bowls, leashes, and collars, a vast array of pet focused accessories such as dog goggles, sun glasses, jewelry, designer clothing and footwear, as well as strollers and backpacks that eliminate the animal's need to walk. In addition, these pet products we now see a growing number of services that cater to the companion animal, such as doggie spas, and chiropractic, massage, laser and acupuncture treatments.

Some of these changes are potentially beneficial to companion animal health, such as advances in pet nutrition and medical treatment (Fox & Gee, 2016). The developments in the pet food industry have been pronounced, resulting in a seemingly never-ending assortment of available options available in flavors, costs, protein sources, breed and size specific requirements, grain content, or level of processing. Veterinary medicine has advanced by leaps and bounds and now includes specialized treatments for preventing or treating serious diseases that were previously considered non-treatable in pets. As a result, companion animals are now living longer than ever before and are following human trends in diseases of aging and obesity.

Not surprisingly, what it means to be a responsible pet owner has evolved in recent years as well (Fox & Gee, 2016). Today's owners feel social pressure to care—to be seen to care—for their pet appropriately and to have a well-behaved and well-controlled animal. In years past, people would commonly let their dogs run free, but leash laws are now common in urban environments; similarly, dog walkers are expected to clean up after their pets. The demand on animal behaviorists to help with training issues has risen, with pet ownership now seen as more "civilized" and integrated into human society.

## Social Capital

Part of understanding this evolving human-animal relationship and its impact at the societal level is to appreciate the degree to which pets confer social capital to their owners or to the people with whom they interact. In other words, what benefits accrue to society from pet ownership and interaction? Companion animals appear to have a number of societal ripple effects that result in improved social capital—the social networks and interactions that inspire trust and reciprocity among citizens (Bulsara, Wood, Giles-Corti, & Bosch, 2007). Pets have been reported to enhance social connections and communication between people in a number of ways. (1) They facilitate social contact and interaction. People report meeting and chatting with others while they are out walking their dogs. They point to the dog as something of "leveler" in that qualities that might otherwise matter to people upon first meeting (e.g., race, wealth, religion, political affiliation, or gender), don't matter as much, and the conversation can safely focus on the dog. (2) Pets facilitate reciprocity via the exchange of pet related favors that build good will and trust. For example, a pet owner may ask a neighbor to watch their dog or cat while they are away. Survey results show that pet owners are also more likely to agree with the statement: "People are willing to help one another". (3) Pets foster civic engagement. For example, dog owners report picking up trash, including discarded items such as used syringes, or the excrement of other dogs while they are out on walks. (4) Pets facilitate an overall sense of community and social capital. Seeing people "out and about" walking their dogs has the downstream ripple effect of creating a sense of community in which people are likely to stop and chat with the dog walkers or with other neighbors that are also outside in their own neighborhoods. (5) Pet ownership, particularly dog ownership, facilitates feelings of safety. A person walking a dog in their own neighborhood is often perceived very much like a roving neighborhood watch. Routine dog walkers are likely to see and notice unusual neighborhood activity and report it. Conversely, seeing people out walking dogs can project a sense of security, suggesting that if there are other people moving around the neighborhood must be safe.

A telephone survey was conducted in four cities, one in Australia (Perth) and three in the United States (San Diego, Portland, and Nashville), with more than 630 residents randomly selected in each city (Wood et al., 2015). Of the pet owners in the sample, over 50% in each city reported that they had gotten to know people in their neighborhood a direct result of their pet. Dog owners were five times more likely than owners of other pets to have gotten to know people in their neighborhood, and those dog owners who walked their dogs were most likely to have neighborhood connections. Further, about one quarter of pet owners who came to know people in their neighborhood through their pets, consider those people to be their friends.

Owning a pet, compared to not owning a pet, has been significantly associated with higher ratings of social capital, and this benefit is not confined to dog owners (Wood et al., 2017). Owners of other pets also rate their levels of social capital to be higher than non-pet owners. It is possible that owning a pet of any kind is linked to perceptions of trust, which is a central component of social capital. Further, it is also possible that pet owners of any kind experience a rise in oxytocin, which is a hormone associated with increased feelings of trust, which may in turn lead pet owners to experience higher levels of social capital. Today, arguably more than ever before, the importance of social connections, tolerance, and trust, cannot be underestimated or undervalued and the research is showing us a key connection between pet ownership and social capital.

## Cultural Considerations

It is difficult to fully understand and consider the human-animal bond or relationship outside of cultural influences. Unfortunately, cultural and other contextual differences such as religion and social class remain poorly understood (Melson & Fine, 2019). For example, we are aware that there is great cultural variation in views about animals and in the practice of keeping pets, and also that there within a given culture there is wide variation in these things, but we know very little about how any individual's background and beliefs may interact with the therapeutic efficacy of human-animal interaction.

As noted by Jegatheesan (2019), the effects of acculturation are not predictable, creating challenges for providers of AAI to anticipate how any individual will respond. Children, for instance, may be influenced by books, television and movies to be more receptive to companion animals than parents who have not been exposed to the same influences. By contrast, individuals who seem to have completely adapted to the values of an adopted culture may nevertheless retain deeply ingrained beliefs about companion animals, stemming from their native religion or culture.

Ethnicity is an important factor related to pet relationships and feelings of neighborhood connectivity (Arkow, 2019). We know that pet keeping is a cross-cultural activity, but very little data exists on the numbers of pets kept by various ethnic groups. However, there is evidence suggesting that the rates of pet keeping are lower among minority populations and specifically in urban communities. It is possible that these individuals are at a greater risk of poverty, unemployment, violent crime and environmental degradation (Arkow, 2019), all of which are likely to make pet ownership less desirable or feasible. It is also important to note that some breeds of dogs, or physical characteristics of those dogs, may have negative cultural associations such as fear or danger which will impact perceptions of those animals (Macnamara, Moga, & Pachel, 2019).

In addition to cultural considerations there are a range of issues related to personal differences that should be weighed when considering an animal-assisted interaction or intervention. Some people simply do not like animals in general, or may prefer only certain types of animals, while others may be fearful of animals, or allergic to certain species. It is important to account for individual preferences, since, for example, a person who is drawn only to cats is unlikely to benefit from an interaction with dogs or horses. Further, some individuals have very specific preferences within a species and may be drawn only to non-shedding dog breeds like Poodles while others may only care for large breeds such as Great Danes and still others prefer small lapdogs like Shitzus. Aside from species or breed preferences the activity level of the animal may be an important consideration. Children often enjoy interacting with rambunctious puppies or kittens, while older adults may prefer the more sedentary or predictable mature companion animal. In all of these cases, considering whether an animal is suited to the individual or situation is paramount, and then if the inclusion of a companion animal appears to be a good match, we must consider the animal's perspective on the situation.

## The Needs of the Animal

A critical topic that we touched upon briefly in several of the preceding chapters is the issue of animal welfare. A fundamental theme running through this text is the importance of making sure that the needs of the animal are not only met, but that the animal enjoys a good quality of life. To accomplish this, it is important to understand species-specific needs and behaviors. Since most animal-assisted interactions tend to involve dogs, we will focus on dogs as the example for our discussion, but it is important to note that other species (e.g., horses, cats, or guinea pigs) will likely have very different nutritional, health, and housing requirements and will need to express very different behaviors in order to experience a good quality of life.

We recommend the following five points as essential to, but not all inclusive of, insuring safety of implementation, and assuring the dog's welfare and quality of life in animal assisted interactions:

1. *Objective Evaluation and Monitoring*—it can be challenging for a dog owner to be objective about their own animal and may push their dog up to or beyond their limits in order to achieve the goals of the activity or program. When this happens, the owner is often trying to run the last subject in a study, or to finish the intervention, or meet a time deadline, with their focus on a number of external pressures and not on the needs of the dog. There are two ways to address this concern: (1) include only registered volunteer therapy dog teams in the activity or intervention. For example, Pet Partners (www.petpartners.org) specifically trains their volunteers to focus on the best interests of their own animals via their YAYABA—You Are Your Animal's Best Advocate training. This allows the practitioner to focus on implementation and external pressures and leaves the volunteer handler free to focus on the needs of their own animal. (2) Implement recommended standards of practice (which typically specify maximum working hours and breaks, among other things) and include a regular schedule of evaluation or observation by a person who is well-suited to the task. A good example of well-established standards of practice is the implementation of the Virginia Commonwealth School of Medicine Dogs on Call program. The organization and implementation of this program has been well documented (Barker, Vokes, & Barker, 2019) and includes regularly scheduled "shadowings" as part of the program. "Shadowings" involve having a disinterested person who has been specifically trained in therapy dog visits with vulnerable populations (in this case hospital patients) to follow and observe a therapy dog team as they proceed through the hospital visitation process. They provide feedback to the handler/dog team and recommend suspension of visits and/or additional training when necessary. This practice insures treatment fidelity and safety for all.
2. *Understanding and Monitoring Signs of Stress in Dogs*—even if another person is responsible for monitoring the dog, it is critical that everyone involved in implementing an animal-assisted activity or intervention understands signs of stress in dogs. Having a number of educated eyes in the environment is the best way to assure detection of the signs of stress in the dog, so that action may be

taken to remove the dog from the stressor. Gee, Hurley, and Rawlings (2016) provide a detailed discussion of the animal's perspective along with number of helpful resources to identifying signs of canine stress and best practices for the inclusion of dogs in animal-assisted interactions. It is essential that the dog is removed from the stressor well before the its stress level escalates to the point of aggressive behavior.

3. *Planning and Preparation*—it is important to plan in advance and to prepare all aspects of introducing a dog into an environment. Coordinate with volunteers about where they may walk their dogs and which doors they may use to enter a building. Take the time to investigate these areas and pathways to determine if they are safe for the dog. It is helpful to avoid high traffic areas if possible, because the likelihood that other people will stop the handler and dog to interact with them can delay the team's timely arrival; this experience may also stress the dog if, for example, a crowd of children rushes to pet them all at once.

4. *Permission*—make sure that you have all required permissions in place to bring a dog into a building. Therapy dogs do not have ADA protection and are only allowed into public buildings with permission of the administration/leadership team. Make sure that others are aware that a dog will be in the area, and when in confined spaces it is important to ask everyone if they are comfortable with the dog entering the space. For example, before getting onto an elevator, ask the occupants if they mind the dog entering the elevator car. Don't assume that everyone wants to interact with the dog and be sure to ask each person if they would like to greet the dog before allowing the dog to approach. When children are involved it is important to get parental consent prior to initiating any dog related activity or intervention, and to ask the child to provide their assent as well. If the child declines by word or action, that should be interpreted as a no, and the dog should not be allowed to approach the child.

5. *Fit for Purpose*—does the dog display appropriate behaviors and indications that demonstrate their ability and desire to work in the environment and with the population of interest? Not all dogs are suited for all tasks; a really good example of this is that some dogs simply are not comfortable around children. Take care to objectively observe the dog's behavior to assess whether it is suited for the task. In best of all worlds, the dog would be assessed by an animal behaviorist, but short of that, another form of objective assessment is key. This requires an evaluation by an impartial individual with a good working knowledge of the signs of stress in dogs.

## Understanding Pet Ownership

There is now an accumulation of evidence indicating a number of ways that pet ownership, particularly dog ownership, has been associated with positive health outcomes (Gee & Mueller, 2019; Kramer, Mehmood, & Suen, 2019). Dog ownership has been associated with decreased risk of cardiovascular disease (Levine et al., 2013), lower blood pressure, improved lipid profile, lower sympathetic response to stress, and lower risk of death (Kramer et al., 2019). What researchers struggle to separate out is whether acquiring a dog makes people healthier, or if healthier people are more likely to acquire a dog? Research on pet ownership is challenging, because people like to choose their own pets, and are not likely to want a researcher to randomly assign a specific pet to them (e.g., dog, cat, or guinea pig), or assign them to be in the no-pet condition of the study. Because of this tendency, a selection bias exists in almost all of the research on the topic of pet ownership, so we have to interpret the findings with caution.

A very small number of studies have managed to overcome these challenges. Pets were randomly assigned to 24 hypertensive stockbrokers, who also received ACE inhibitors (Allen, Shykoff, & Izzo, 2001). A control group of the same size and characteristics received ACE inhibitors only. At the beginning of the study both groups demonstrated the same cardiovascular responses to mental stress; after 6 months, the blood pressure responses of the pet owning group were significantly reduced, allowing for a reduction or removal of medication for the treatment of hypertension.

Looking at psychological, rather than physical, Ko, Youn, Kim, and Kim (2016) randomly assigned each of 46 community dwelling Korean older adults to care for five caged crickets over a period of eight weeks. When comparing results of psychometric and laboratory tests taken at baseline and repeated at the conclusion of the study, the cricket-caring group showed reduced depression and improved cognition when compared with a control group ($N = 48$).

Although some people favor the idea of prescribing pets as a treatment for certain diseases (e.g., depression), or conditions (e.g., loneliness), or as a way of improving health, the evidence is not strong enough, yet, to support these sorts of prescriptions. In fact, prescribing a pet for the treatment of a disease is currently problematic for a number of reasons. First, such a prescription may be interpreted by the patient, as something they should do instead of seeking professional help or embarking on an evidence-based treatment or medication plan. Second, people who are suffering from a disease may not be in a position, physically, mentally, or financially, to care for the needs of the animal. Third, medical professionals may or may not be aware of species-specific needs or behaviors and may not have the working knowledge to match the person with the most appropriate animal or breed of animal. Fourth, prescribing a pet will require follow-up by a trained professional and it is unclear what type of individual would be appropriate to follow up with the patient while at the same time overseeing the welfare of the animal. With all of that said, it is entirely possible that companion animals can, and will be, prescribed by healthcare professionals someday, but as is the case with all remedies prescribed by doctors, much research needs to be done to establish efficacy and dosage, to insure treatment fidelity and in this case, animal welfare.

## Establishing the Evidence Base

The field of human-animal interaction research, also known as Anthrozoology, has historically been plagued by low quality research methodology (Kazdin, 2017) and a positive publication bias (Herzog, Podberscek, & Docherty, 2005). Much of the early research relied on small sample sizes which were unlikely to represent the larger population of people who own or interact with animals. Additionally, those studies often reflected anecdotal reports, descriptive case-studies, or studies without controls, or used correlational methods that did not allow for causal attributions. In other words, these reports frequently provided detailed examples or information about how various attributes of human-animal interaction were related, but fell short in establishing causal links or understanding underlying mechanisms of action. The field is also probably more prone than other fields toward a positive publication bias simply because there are so many animal-lovers who enjoy reading about the many ways that pets may be good for people. It is not uncommon to see a heartwarming pet-related story in newspapers, magazines, television news broadcasts, social media, or other form of popular press.

In order to fully establish the evidence base fundamental to human-animal interaction, as researchers we need to take several steps

1. *Fully Develop and Test Theories*—to understand the mechanisms of action underlying the importance, the impact, and the nature, of the human-animal bond those mechanisms must be proposed in detail and tested specifically. To accomplish this, clearly defined and stated theories need to be developed, and tested, and refined, and tested again. This iterative process is fundamental to scientific exploration and understanding. We are at the precipice of describing and predicting the nature of the human-animal bond, but theory is required to move forward.
2. *Ask Good Questions*—the questions asked by researchers shape the answers they find in doing research. We need to understand the ways in which animals may effect change in various aspects of the human condition. At the same time, we need to understand the how, when, where, and why these changes may take place. In order to establish an evidence base indicative of the value and efficacy of companion animal interaction or ownership we need to ask relevant questions that provide the opportunity to disprove the popular notion that animals are always beneficial.
3. *Use a Wide Variety of High-Quality Research Methodologies*—to fully establish an evidence base a wide variety of research methodologies need to be employed to help researchers better understand the how, when, where and why of animal interaction or ownership. Descriptive techniques and qualitative research are important to fully understand the many subtle and important variables that may be involved, or that need to be controlled, or that need to be treated as potential confounders in more sophisticated research designs. Ultimately, however, we need empirical research using randomized controlled trials to establish causal links. In other words, we need to randomly assigned conditions so that we can say with more confidence whether a particular treatment (e.g., interaction

with an animal) causes specific health outcomes to change (e.g., decreases in cardiovascular disease).
4. *Longitudinal Approach*—it isn't enough to find that owning, or interacting with, an animal causes a short-term change in any particular health outcome; we need to see if that change is sustained over time. In order to accomplish this, we need to study the effects of pet ownership or interaction over time. People tend to own pets for many years, and even if we find that pets are good for people at any particular point in time, we cannot assume that the pet will always have the same effect. The needs and behaviors of people change over time, as do the needs and behaviors of pets. What may be beneficial to a person at the age of 20 may be very different for someone aged 3, or 80. Likewise a dog at the age of 3 is likely behave very differently from a dog at the age of 12 weeks or 12 years. The relationship between pets and people is dynamic and likely to be complicated by health changes in the person or the pet, or both. For example, having a pet that unwell can be immensely stressful to a human. Likewise, a person who is injured or ill may not be able to adequately care for their pet; omitting routine activities, such as long walks, can be stressful on the pet.
5. *Large Sample Sizes*—to fully represent the broad range of people who may benefit from companion animal ownership or interaction, we must include large representative samples of people of all ages, and from all walks of life. Further, to fully understand the potential impact afforded by the wide variety of animals maintained as pets, we need research that focuses on many different species and within species, on the diversity of breeds.
6. *Determine dosage and best fit*—the idea of dosage refers to how much time one needs to spend with a companion animal in a particular activity or situation in order to accrue any potential benefits. The idea of best fit refers to the best pairing between companion animals and people to the maximum and mutual benefit of both.

In this volume we have defined human well-being and described how it evolves or varies over the life course, briefly reviewed the research on human-animal interactions, and discussed how pets may play a role in the family life cycle, in human health over the life course, in child health and development, and in aging populations. Additionally, we have described a broad spectrum of animal assisted interventions and how an aging pet may impact well-being. Here in the conclusion we have brought these topics together and also taken a step back to view the bigger picture. We have examined the changing conceptions of pet ownership and interactions in recent years, the effect of pets on social capital, the impact of cultural and individual differences in relation to companion animals, the animal's perspective on human-animal interactions, and various ways we must meet the needs of the animals involved. We discussed the existing evidence and the difficulties associated with studying pet ownership as a variable, and finally we make recommendations for next steps in establishing the evidence base.

There is much to do, but this short discussion of the existing evidence indicates that there is something to this human-animal bond. There is reason to continue to investigate the impact of companion animals on human-health and well-being and the future is bright for those interesting in studying human-animal interaction and those interested in practicing animal-assisted interventions. We are on the edge of developing a greater understanding of the human-animal bond and of vastly improving implementations of animal-assisted interventions such that both species may benefit maximally from these interactions.

# References

Allen, K., Shykoff, B. E., & Izzo, J. L., Jr. (2001). Pet ownership, but not ACE inhibitor therapy, blunts home blood pressure responses to mental stress. *Hypertension, 38*(4), 815–820.

Arkow, P. (2019). The social capital of companion animals: Pets as a catalyst for social networks and support… and a barometer of community violence. In *Handbook on animal-assisted therapy* (pp. 51–60). San Diego: Academic Press.

Barker, S. B., Vokes, R. A., & Barker, R. T. (2019). *Animal-Assisted Interventions in Health Care Settings: A best practice manual for establishing new programs*. West Lafayette, IN: Purdue University Press.

Bulsara, M., Wood, L., Giles-Corti, B., & Bosch, D. (2007). More than a furry companion: The ripple effect of companion animals on neighborhood interactions and sense of community. *Society & Animals, 15*(1), 43–56.

Fox, R., & Gee, N. R. (2016). Changing conceptions of care: Humanization of the companion animal-human relationship. *Society & Animals, 24*(2), 107–128.

Gee, N. R., Hurley, K. J., & Rawlings, J. M. (2016). From the dog's perspective: Welfare implications of HAI research and practice.

Gee, N. R., & Mueller, M. K. (2019). A systematic review of research on pet ownership and animal interactions among older adults. *Anthrozoös, 32*(2), 183–207.

Herzog, H. A., Podberscek, A. L., & Docherty, A. (2005). The reliability of peer review in anthrozoology. *Anthrozoös, 18,* 175–182.

Jegatheesan, B. (2019). Influence of cultural and religious factors on attitudes toward animals. In *handbook on animal-assisted therapy* (pp. 43–50). San Diego: Academic Press.

Kazdin, A. E. (2017). *Research design in clinical psychology*. Boston, MA: Pearson.

Ko, H. J., Youn, C. H., Kim, S. H., & Kim, S. Y. (2016). Effect of pet insects on the psychological health of community-dwelling elderly people: A single-blinded, randomized, controlled trial. *Gerontology, 62,* 200–209.

Kramer, C. K., Mehmood, S., & Suen, R. S. (2019). Dog ownership and survival: A systematic review and meta-analysis. *Circulation: Cardiovascular Quality and Outcomes, 12*(10).

Levine, G. N., Allen, K., Braun, L. T., Christian, H. E., Friedmann, E., Taubert, K. A., et al. (2013). Pet ownership and cardiovascular risk: A scientific statement from the American Heart Association. *Circulation, 127,* 2353–2363.

Macnamara, M., Moga J., Pachel, C. (2019). What's love got to do with it? Selecting animals for animal-assisted mental health interventions. In *Handbook on animal-assisted therapy* (pp. 43–50). San Diego: Academic Press.

Melson, G. F., Fine, A. H. (2019). Animals in the Lives of Children. In *Handbook on Animal-Assisted Therapy* (pp. 249–269). Academic Press.

Wood, L., Martin, K., Christian, H., Houghton, S., Kawachi, I., Vallesi, S., & McCune, S. (2017). Social capital and pet ownership—A tale of four cities. *SSM-population health, 3,* 442.

Wood, L., Martin, K., Christian, H., Nathan, A., Lauritsen, C., Houghton, S., … McCune, S. (2015). The pet factor-companion animals as a conduit for getting to know people, friendship formation and social support. *PloS one, 10*(4).

**Nancy R. Gee, Ph.D.** is Professor of Psychiatry, Bill Balaban Chair of Human-Animal Interaction, and Director of the Center for Human-Animal Interaction in the School of Medicine at Virginia Commonwealth University. Previously Dr. Gee served as the Human-Animal Interaction Research Manager, for the Waltham Petcare Science Institute in Leicestershire England. She has published extensively on HAI, including her most recent book; *How Animals Help Students Learn: Research and Practice for Educators and Mental-Health Professionals.* Dr. Gee continues to pursue research in HAI across the lifespan, seeking to identify the ways in which interactions with companion animals affect human cognition, mental, and physical health. Concern for the animal's welfare and quality of life is a primary consideration for Dr. Gee, both in the Dogs on Call hospital visitation program she administers and in her various research and writing projects. Dr. Gee is a recipient of multiple grants and awards, a member of several organizational boards and journal editorial advisory boards, reviewer of HAI research grant proposals, and frequent presenter at national and international HAI conferences.

GPSR Compliance
The European Union's (EU) General Product Safety Regulation (GPSR) is a set of rules that requires consumer products to be safe and our obligations to ensure this.

If you have any concerns about our products, you can contact us on

ProductSafety@springernature.com

In case Publisher is established outside the EU, the EU authorized representative is:

Springer Nature Customer Service Center GmbH
Europaplatz 3
69115 Heidelberg, Germany

www.ingramcontent.com/pod-product-compliance
Ingram Content Group UK Ltd.
Pitfield, Milton Keynes, MK11 3LW, UK
UKHW020037040925
462575UK00012B/431